Otitis Media: State of the Art Concepts and Treatment

Diego Preciado
Editor

Otitis Media: State of the Art Concepts and Treatment

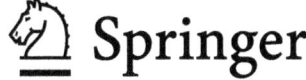 Springer

Editor
Diego Preciado
Department of Pediatric Otolaryngology
Children's National Medical Center
Washington
District of Columbia
USA

ISBN 978-3-319-17887-5   ISBN 978-3-319-17888-2 (eBook)
DOI 10.1007/978-3-319-17888-2

Library of Congress Control Number: 201594228

Springer Cham Heidelberg New York Dordrecht London

Printed on acid-free paper

Springer is a brand of Springer International Publishing
Springer International Publishing is part of Springer Science+Business Media (www.springer.com)

Contents

Part III   Treatments

Contributors

Jill Arganbright Otolaryngology, Children's Mercy Hospital and Clinics, Kansas City, MO, USA

Lauren O. Bakaletz Department of Pediatrics, The Research Institute at Nationwide Children's Hospital, Ohio State University College of Medicine, Columbus, OH, USA

Margaretha L. Casselbrant Division of Pediatric Otolaryngology, Children's Hospital of Pittsburgh of UPMC, Pittsburgh, PA, USA

Department of Otolaryngology, University of Pittsburgh School of Medicine, Pittsburgh, PA, USA

Jonathan Cavanagh Department of Surgery, Janeway Children's Hospital, St John's, Canada

Craig Derkay Department of Otolaryngology Head Neck Surgery, Eastern Virginia Medical School, Children's Hospital of the King's Daughters, Norfolk, VA, USA

Ximena Fonseca Department of Otolaryngology, Head and Neck Surgery, Hospital Clinico Pontificia Universidad Catolica De Chile, Santiago, Chile

Shannon Fraser Department of Otolaryngology, University of Pittsburgh School of Medicine, Pittsburgh, PA, USA

Ricardo Godinho Department of Medicine, Medical School Pontifical Catholic University of Minas Gerais, Sete Lagoas, MG, Brazil

Christopher R. Grindle Division of Otolaryngology—Head and Neck Surgery, University of Connecticut School of Medicine, Hartford, CT, USA

Jennifer Ha Department of Otolaryngology Head and Neck Surgery, Perth Children's Hospital, Subiaco, WA, Australia

Peggy Kelley Otolaryngology, Children's Hospital Colorado, Aurora, CO, USA

Rita Krumenaur Department of Pediatric Otolaryngology, Santo Antonio Hospital for Children, Porto Alegre, Brazil

Jizhen Lin Department of Otolaryngology, University of Minnesota Hospitals and Clinics, Minneapolis, MN, USA

José Faibes Lubianca Neto Department of Otolaryngology and Pediatric Otorhinolaryngology, Santo Antônio Childrens Hospital, Porto Alegre, RS, Brazil

Laura A. Novotny Department of Pediatrics, The Research Institute at Nationwide Children's Hospital, Center for Microbial Pathogensis, Columbus, OH, USA

J. Christopher Post Departments of Surgery and Microbiology, Allegheny General Hospital, Pittsburgh, PA, USA

Temple University School of Medicine and Drexel University College of Medicine, Pittsburgh, PA, USA

Diego Preciado Division of Pediatric Otolaryngology, Children's National Medical Center, Washington, DC, USA

Sarah Prunty Department of Otolaryngology Head and Neck Surgery, Perth Children's Hospital, Subiaco, WA, Australia

Amanda G. Ruiz Otolaryngology, The University of Colorado School of Medicine, Children's Hospital Colorado, Aurora, CO, USA

José San Martín Department of Otolaryngology, Head and Neck Surgery, Hospital Clinico Pontificia Universidad Catolica De Chile, Santiago, Chile

Tania Sih Department of Pediatric Otolaryngology, Medical School University of São Paulo, São Paulo, Brazil

Stéphanie Val Sheikh Zayed Institute, The Otologic Laboratory, Children's National Health System, Center for Genetic Medicine Research, Washington, DC, USA

Shyan Vijayasekaran Department of Otolaryngology Head and Neck Surgery, Perth Children's Hospital, Subiaco, WA, Australia

Lyndy Wilcox Department of Otolaryngology Head Neck Surgery, Eastern Virginia Medical School, Children's Hospital of the King's Daughters, Norfolk, VA, USA

Audie Woolley Department of Otolaryngology and Pediatrics, The Children's Hospital of Alabama, Birmingham, AL, USA

Part I
Introduction

Otitis Media Concepts, Facts, and Fallacies

Diego Preciado

Introduction

Otitis media (OM) is the most common diagnosis for medical visits in preschool-age children [1] and the most frequent indication for outpatient antibiotic use in the USA and the world, with estimated annual public health cost totaling US$ 2.8 billion annually [2, 3]. OM is characterized by signs and symptoms of middle-ear effusion (MEE), by definition fluid collection in the middle ear. It may also include otorrhea (drainage of fluid from the middle ear), which occurs after perforation of the tympanic membrane™ or through ventilation tubes placed previously.

Even though the disease is characterized by a tremendously widespread prevalence, deep-rooted and significant controversies still exist regarding its diagnosis, pathophysiology, and medical and surgical management. Medical literature on the subject is strewn across multiple medical disciplines; as such it is difficult to stay up-to-date on a majority of the reported advances. Importantly, over the past 13 years, there has been a modest but steady decrease in US pediatric encounter rates for OM, with 4.6% fewer outpatient encounters and 9.8% fewer hospital discharges [3]. This represents a reversal of a previously reported long-term increasing trend and is thought to be primarily attributable to decreased secondhand smoke exposure and to widespread bacterial and viral vaccination efforts.

Definitions

OM can be classified as: acute otitis media (AOM), otitis media with effusion (OME), recurrent AOM, and chronic suppurative OM (CSOM). Each will have a separate basis in its best course of treatment.

AOM is defined by the presence of middle-ear inflammation and fluid of sudden onset and often presents with constitutional symptoms consistent with infection, such as fever and pain. OME is characterized by MEE without otalgia, fever, and distinct signs of ongoing inflammation typical of AOM. Recurrent AOM is defined as three or more AOM episodes occurring in the previous 6 months or four or more AOM episodes in the preceding 12 months. OME that persists beyond 3 months is called chronic OM or chronic OME.

CSOM is different from chronic OME and is defined as purulent otorrhea associated with a chronic tympanic membrane™ perforation that persists for more than 6 weeks despite appropriate treatment for AOM.

D. Preciado (✉)
Division of Pediatric Otolaryngology, Children's
National Medical Center, Washington, DC 20010, USA
e-mail: dpreciad@cnmc.org

© Springer International Publishing Switzerland 2015
D. Preciado (ed.), *Otitis Media: State of the art concepts and treatment*, DOI 10.1007/978-3-319-17888-2_1

Epidemiology and Risk Factors

Age

The incidence of OM decreases steadily as the age of a child increases. Epidemiologic studies reveal the peak rate of infections occurring in patients between 6 and 18 months [4]. This is likely reflective of increased maturity of the immune system and completion of childhood vaccinations. A decrease is also observed as the anatomy of the eustachian tube changes with craniofacial maturation, which will be further discussed in another section.

Risk factors for OM propensity include host, environmental, and pathogen-related factors. As such, OM is a multifactorial condition. Risk factors for OM susceptibility will be discussed in detail in a separate chapter.

Pathogenesis

Clearly a multifactorial disease process, risk profile, and host-pathogen interactions have increasingly become recognized as playing important roles in the pathogenesis of OM. Such events as alterations in mucociliary clearance through repeated viral exposure experienced in daycare settings or through exposure to tobacco smoke may tip the balance of pathogenesis in less virulent OM pathogens in their favor, especially in children with a unique host predisposition.

AOM typically occurs after an infection that results in increased congestion of the nasopharynx and eustachian tube. When increased secretions are present, the eustachian tube becomes obstructed and creates persistent negative pressures within the middle ear. Over time, the alteration in pressure can result in reflux of nasopharyngeal contents into the middle ear. Negative pressure also can cause increased vascular permeability and can lead to the development of an effusion. In AOM, the effusion contains microorganisms that proliferate in the middle ear and lead to classic acute symptomatology.

Eustachian Tube Anatomy

Studies of patients born with craniofacial abnormalities provide evidence to the role of Eustachian Tube (ET) maturation in the pathogenesis of OM. Histologic studies of ET tissue from children born with cleft lip or palate show evidence of immaturity of the cartilaginous tissue of the tube, which may explain the higher propensity toward infection in those children. Similarly, imaging studies demonstrate a more horizontal orientation of the tube, allowing for more direct entry of bacteria into the middle ear.

Microbiology

The three most common cultured bacteria responsible for infection are *Streptococcus pneumoniae, Haemophilus influenzae,* and *Moraxella catarrhalis.* Historically, the role of *S. pneumoniae* is well established; it was first described as the cause of OM in 1888. These bacteria are not routine colonizers in the external auditory canal (EAC) but are frequently found in the nasopharynx, which further supports the mechanism of infection [5]. The majority of infections are caused by *S. pneumoniae* or *H. influenzae,* and there is regional variation in the most common pathogen. Clinical evidence indicates that *S. pneumoniae* is a more virulent pathogen in the middle ear and is more often recovered from recurrent cases of AOM or after treatment failures. Some studies have found that *S. pneumoniae* infection can lead to a higher fever and more toxic appearance of the patient [6]. However, there are no known otoscopic differences between those pathogens.

H. influenzae is frequently isolated from the nasopharynx. Faden et al. found that nearly half of studied children carried the bacteria [7]. Prior to the availability of the *H. influenzae* type b vaccine series, approximately 10% of cases were due to typable Haemophilus b strains. Currently, non-typable *H. influenzae* (NTHi) is the most common pathogen isolated in AOM cases. Moraxella species are also common colonizers of the nasopharynx in children and infants. Interestingly, cases of OM in which *M. catarrhalis* was isolated were rare until the 1980s.

Group A Streptococci, Staphylococcus aureus, and gram-negative bacilli are responsible for the minority of infections. Isolation of *S. aureus* or *Pseudomonas aeruginosa* in particular may indicate an underlying systemic disease such as HIV or diabetes. Group A species, more often found in cases of pharyngitis, may cause OM through direct alteration of the eustachian tube function. However, it is currently not a significant pathogen.

Bacterial Resistance Patterns

Children <2 years of age in regular contact with large groups of other children, especially in daycare settings, or who recently have received antimicrobial treatment are at largest risk for harboring resistant bacteria in the nasopharynx and middle-ear space. Many strains of each of the abovementioned pathogenic bacteria that commonly cause AOM are resistant to commonly used antimicrobial drugs.

Although antimicrobial resistance rates vary across the globe, in the USA approximately 40% of strains of NTHi and a great majority of *M. catarrhalis* strains are resistant to aminopenicillins (e.g., ampicillin and amoxicillin). For these organisms, the resistance is attributable to production of β-lactamase against the penicillin molecule, which may be overcome by combining amoxicillin with a β-lactamase inhibitor (clavulanate) or by using a β-lactamase-stable antibiotic. It is worth noting that bacterial resistance rates in northern European countries where antibiotic usage is less are comparatively exceedingly lower (β -lactamase resistance in 6–10% of isolates) than in the US.

In the USA, approximately 50% of strains of *S. pneumoniae* are penicillin-nonsusceptible, divided approximately equally between penicillin-intermediate and, even more difficult to treat, penicillin-resistant strains. As opposed to NTHi and *M. catarrhalis,* resistance by *S. pneumoniae* to the penicillins and other β-lactam antibiotics

is mediated not by β-lactamase production, but almost exclusively due to alterations in penicillin-binding proteins, which are overcome not by adding β-lactamase inhibitors, but by increasing the dosage of the penicillin-based antibiotic and increasing the local concentration of the drug in the middle-ear space. In general, as penicillin resistance increases, so also does resistance to other antimicrobial classes. Resistance to macrolides, including azithromycin and clarithromycin, by *S. pneumoniae* has increased rapidly, rendering theses antimicrobials minimally effective in AOM.

Diagnosis

Accurate diagnosis of OM presents a diagnostic challenge, yet, appropriate use of diagnostic criteria is essential to prevent complications, while minimizing overuse of antibiotics. As opposed to the 2004 guidelines from the American Academy of Pediatrics and the American Academy of Family Practice, the 2013 guidelines now include diagnostic accuracy as an essential component of treatment approaches [8]. Typically, otoscopy may reveal loss of bony landmarks, bulging eardrum or poor mobility of the tympanic membrane (TM).

Current literature indicates that pneumatic otoscopy is the most accurate method of diagnosis when used by an experienced clinician. However, routine use in clinical practice is variable, and the accuracy of the diagnosis may be dependent on the comfort of the examiner [9]. It is important to note that the sensitivity and specificity of this technique applies only to pneumatic otoscopy, not otoscopy alone. Commonly used diagnostic criteria such as erythema of the TM may be nonspecific signs of fever or crying.

Tympanometry

Tympanometry is a complementary exam to otoscopy that aims to determine the resistance (impedance) of the middle-ear system. A sound probe is inserted into the ear canal, and sound pressure (at 226 Hz typically) is presented into the ear canal while altering air pressure of the external ear canal from +200 to −400 decapascal (daPa). Under normal conditions, there will be a peak that is elicited, with the ear drum "moving" upon the change in pressure. The volume of the ear canal can be directly inferred and automatically recorded from the measured compliance of the middle-ear system. Tympanograms may be grouped into 1 of 3 categories. Tracings characterized by a relatively steep gradient, sharp-angled peak, and middle-ear air pressure (location of the peak in terms of air pressure) that approximates atmospheric pressure (type A curve) are assumed to indicate normal middle-ear status. Tracings characterized by a shallow peak or no peak and by negative or indeterminate middle-ear air pressure are often termed "flat" or type B and are usually assumed to indicate the presence of a middle-ear abnormality that is causing decreased TM compliance. The most common such abnormality, by far, in infants and children is MEE. Tracings characterized by intermediate findings—somewhat shallow peak, often in association with a gradual gradient (obtuse-angled peak) or negative middle-ear air pressure peak (often termed type 'C') or combinations of these features—may or may not be associated with MEE and must be considered nondiagnostic or equivocal. In general, the shallower the peak, the more gradual the gradient, and the more negative the middle-ear air pressure, the greater the likelihood of MEE.

When reading a tympanogram, it is important to look at the volume measurement. The type B tympanometric response has to be analyzed within the context of the recorded volume. A flat, 'low' volume (1 mL or less) tracing typically reflects the volume of the ear canal only, representing MEE, which impedes the movement of an intact ear drum. A flat, high volume (>1 cc) tracing typically reflects the volume of the ear canal and middle-ear space, representing a perforation (or patent pressure equalization tube) in the tympanic membrane. A patient with a tympanic membrane perforation or patent tympanostomy tube will have a flat type B tympanogram and a "high volume." The tympanometer measures and records the volume of the external auditory canal, and if a tympanic membrane perforation or a pat-

ent tympanostomy tube is present, the volume of the middle ear and mastoid air cells as well. A volume reading >1.0 mL should suggest the presence of either a perforation or a patent tympanostomy tube. Therefore, in a child with a tympanostomy tube present, a flat tympanogram with a volume <1.0 mL would suggest a plugged or nonfunctioning tube and middle-ear fluid, while a flat tympanogram with a volume >1.0 mL would suggest a patent tympanostomy tube.

Tympanocentesis

Tympanocentesis confirms the presence of an effusion. Aspiration of fluid provides a sample for culture so that targeted therapy may be used. Still, tympanocentesis is not performed for routine AOM as empiric treatment or observation often result in improvement of symptoms. The procedure is indicated for treatment failure after two complete courses of empiric antibiotics, sepsis evaluation, mastoiditis, or for patients with immune deficiency. It is also performed in the research setting. Culture data from tympanocentesis provided valuable information on the microbiology of middle-ear infection. In reality, pain and discomfort associated with the condition limit the use of this in routine clinical practice as well.

Acoustic Reflexometry

This method measures changes in the TM that can be correlated with measurement of middle-ear pressure and is useful in diagnosing effusion. The advantage of this technique is that a tight seal is not necessary for proper use. However, this method is currently used in research and is not available in routine clinical use.

Treatment

While the diagnosis of AOM can be complicated, the judicious use of antibiotics in this illness is difficult. Providers must weigh carefully the goal of improved symptoms and prevention of potential complications against overprescribing antibiotics. In strains of *S. pneumoniae,* a number of resistant strains are colonizers in the nasopharynx that circulate in the community. Additionally, development of novel resistant strains is quite rapid [10].

Conservative Management and Observation

In efforts to reduce overuse of antibiotics and minimize unnecessary side effects, the role of careful observation is appealing. By 24 h after diagnosis, 61% of children who have AOM have decreased symptoms, whether they receive placebo or antibiotics, and by 1 week, approximately 75% have resolution of their symptoms [11], it is worthy to mention that younger children or those who demonstrate severe otalgia, bilateral infection, high or persistent fever should not be managed with observation, but should be treated with antibiotics [8]. The most accurate treatment paradigm for antibiotic therapy will be discussed in more detail in a separate chapter, but in general high-dose Amoxicillin (90 mg/kg) remains the first-line option for a majority of cases. Oral cephalosporins such as cefdinir and cefuroxime are effective options for children with sensitivity to Amoxicillin. Amoxicillin-clavulanate also in high dose is recommended for treatment failures (no improvement in 72 h). Intramuscular ceftriaxone can also be given either only once or with a repeat injection 72 h later. Patients who have severe type I allergy to penicillin (PCN) antibiotics should receive a combination of clindamycin (30–40 mg/kg per day in three divided doses) to cover *S. pneumoniae* and sulfisoxazole for non-typable *H. influenzae.* Those patients who have non-type I penicillin allergies should be prescribed oral cephalosporins such as cefdinir (14 mg/kg per day divided twice a day or daily, with twice-daily therapy approved for 5–10 days), cefuroxime (30 mg/kg per day in two divided doses), cefpodoxime (10 mg/kg per day once daily), or intramuscular ceftriaxone (50 mg/kg for 1–3 days). Overall, longer therapy duration

is shown to be more effective at treating acute infection, but does not show long-term benefit in preventing relapse [12]. Tympanocentesis should also be strongly considered for immunocompromised patients, neonates younger than 2 weeks of age, and patients who have AOM that has been refractory to treatment or if AOM is present in infants within the first 2 months of birth to identify the causative organisms and target antibiotic therapy more accurately.

There is no role for the usage of antibiotics in the long-term clearance of chronic middle-ear fluid, and as such they are not indicated in patients with chronic OME.

Surgical Treatment

Myringotomy and Insertion of Tympanostomy Tubes

When AOM is recurrent, despite appropriate medical therapy, consideration of surgical management of AOM with tympanostomy tube insertion is warranted, especially when there is persistent effusion at the time of otolaryngologic evaluation. This procedure has been shown to be highly effective in reducing the rate of AOM in patients with recurrent OM and to significantly improve the quality of life in patients with recurrent AOM. Individual patient factors including risk-profile, severity of AOM episodes, the child's development and age, the presence of a history of adverse drug reactions, concurrent medical problems, and the parental wishes influence decision making in this regard. Importantly, if there is no MEE present at the time of otolaryngologic evaluation, the latest set of guidelines state that surgical tympanostomy tube placement is not indicated.

Post-myringotomy Tube Otorrhea

Although tympanostomy tubes generally greatly reduce the incidence of AOM in most children, patients with tympanostomy tubes may still develop AOM. A clear advantage of tympanostomy tubes in children with recurrent AOM is that if they do develop an episode of AOM with a functioning tube in place, these patients will manifest purulent drainage from the tube. By definition, children with functioning tympanostomy tubes without otorrhea do not have AOM as a cause for a presentation of fever or behavioral changes. If tympanostomy tube otorrhea develops, ototopical treatment should be considered as first-line therapy. With a functioning tube in place, the infection is able to drain, and the possibility of developing a serious complication from an episode of AOM is negligible. The current quinolone otic drops approved by the US Food and Drug Administration for use in the middle-ear space in children are formulated with ciprofloxacin/dexamethasone (Ciprodex) and ofloxacin (Floxin). The topical delivery of these otic drops allows them to utilize a higher concentration than would be tolerated orally and have excellent coverage of even the most resistant strains of common middle-ear pathogens. Suctioning and removal of the secretions, often done through referral to an otolaryngologist, may be quite helpful. When children with tube otorrhea fail to improve satisfactorily with conventional outpatient management, they may require tube removal or hospitalization to receive parenteral antibiotic treatment, or both.

Surgical Treatment for Chronic OME

A full audiological evaluation should be performed for patients with effusions present for >3 months, as most cases of OME resolve without treatment within 3 months after an AOM spell. However, when MEE is present in a patient sporadically, without a clear history of AOM or upper respiratory tract infection, it may be less likely to clear over time [13]. When MEE persists longer than 3 months, consideration of surgical management with tympanostomy tubes is appropriate. In considering the decision to refer the patient for consultation, the clinician should attempt to determine the impact of the OME on the child. Although hearing loss may be of primary concern, OME causes a number of other difficulties in children that should also be considered. These include predisposition to recurring AOM, pain, disturbance of balance, and tinnitus. In addition, long-term sequelae that have been demonstrated to be associated with OME include pathologic middle-ear changes, atelectasis of the tympanic membrane and retraction pocket formation, adhesive OM, cholesteatoma formation and ossicular discontinuity, and conductive and sensorineural hearing loss. Long-term adverse effects on speech, language, cognitive and psychosocial development have also been demonstrated, although some studies have demonstrated that the long-term adverse impact of OME on development may be small in otherwise healthy children. In considering the impact of OME on development, it is especially important to take into consideration the overall presentation of the child. Although it is unlikely that OME causing unilateral hearing loss in the mild range will have long-term negative effects on an otherwise healthy and developmentally normal child, even a mild hearing loss in a child with other developmental or speech delays certainly has the potential to compound this child's difficulties.

This book aims to elaborate on much of what has been mentioned above in this introductory chapter, while also clarifying areas of controversy in OM. Two comprehensive reviews on basic science concepts, role of innate immunity and mucins, inflammatory regulation, and state-of-the-art translational research is also included. Experts on vaccine development for OM prevention also review the latest efforts in this regard. A thorough review of OM complications and of the treatment and management of CSOM will also be included in the second part of the book. Finally, best management paradigms for a unique subset of patients with OM, those with cochlear implants, will be included.

References

1. Schappert SM. Office visits for otitis media: United States, 1975–90. Adv Data. 1992;8:1–19.
2. Stool SE, Field MJ. The impact of otitis media. Pediatr Infect Dis J. 1989;8:11–4.

3. Grubb MS, Spaugh DC. Treatment failure, recurrence, and antibiotic prescription rates for different acute otitis media treatment methods. Clin Pediatr (Phila). 2010;49:970–5.

4. Daly KA, Giebink GS. Clinical epidemiology of otitis media. Pediatr Infect Dis J. 2000;19:31–6.

5. Stenfors LE, Bye HM, Raisanen S. Causes for massive bacterial colonization on mucosal membranes during infectious mononucleosis: implications for acute otitis media. Int J Pediatr Otorhinolaryngol. 2002;65:233–40.

6. Rodriguez WJ, Schwartz RH. *Streptococcus pneumoniae* causes otitis media with higher fever and more redness of tympanic membranes than *Haemophilus influenzae* or *Moraxella catarrhalis*. Pediatr Infect Dis J. 1999;18:942–4.

7. Faden H, Duffy L, Wasielewski R, Wolf J, Krystofik D, Tung Y. Relationship between nasopharyngeal colonization and the development of otitis media in children. Tonawanda/Williamsville Pediatrics. J Infect Dis. 1997;175:1440–5.

8. Lieberthal AS, Carroll AE, Chonmaitree T, et al. The diagnosis and management of acute otitis media. Pediatrics. 2013;131:e964–99.

9. Steinbach WJ, Sectish TC, Benjamin DK Jr, Chang KW, Messner AH. Pediatric residents' clinical diagnostic accuracy of otitis media. Pediatrics. 2002;109:993–8.

10. Dagan R, Leibovitz E, Cheletz G, Leiberman A, Porat N. Antibiotic treatment in acute otitis media promotes superinfection with resistant *Streptococcus pneumoniae* carried before initiation of treatment. J Infect Dis. 2001;183:880–6.

11. Rosenfeld RM, Kay D. Natural history of untreated otitis media. Laryngoscope. 2003;113:1645–57.

12. Cohen R, Levy C, Boucherat M, et al. Five vs. ten days of antibiotic therapy for acute otitis media in young children. Pediatr Infect Dis J. 2000;19:458–63.

13. Rosenfeld RM, Schwartz SR, Pynnonen MA, et al. Clinical practice guideline: tympanostomy tubes in children. Otolaryngol Head Neck Surg. 2013;149:1–35.

Part II
Concepts and Diagnosis

Epidemiology of Otitis Media: What Have We Learned from the New Century Global Health Disparities

2

Ricardo Godinho and Tania Sih

Introduction

Otitis media (OM) is the most frequent reason for which children see a doctor and can be defined as a continuum of conditions that includes acute OM (AOM), OM with residual or persistent effusion, unresponsive OM, recurrent OM (ROM), OM with complications, and chronic OM. The pathogenic mechanisms of OM involve interactions among host characteristics, virulence factors of viral and bacterial pathogens, and environmental factors. A statistical report from the US Agency for Healthcare Research and Quality [1] examined childhood ear infections using the Medical Expenditure Panel Survey 2006 Full Year Consolidated File and showed that the expenditures for outpatient treatment and prescriptions totaled $ 2.8 billion in 2006. Annual hospital discharge rates for OM declined by 73 % as determined from the National Hospital Discharge Survey (NHDS) [2, 3].

The literature has continued to expand, increasing understanding of the worldwide burden of OM in childhood. Population-based studies confirmed reductions in OM prevalence. Although most studies concentrated on AOM or OM with effusion (OME), a few examined severe chronic suppurative OM (CSOM), a major public health problem in developing countries and for certain indigenous populations around the world.

For most children, progression to tympanic membrane perforation and CSOM is unusual (low-risk populations). Yet in some communities, more than 4 % of the children are affected by chronic tympanic membrane perforation with chronic drainage (high-risk populations). In developing countries, where children have limited access to medical care, suppurative complications of OM are frequent with a high risk of permanent hearing loss. In developed countries, the most common morbidity of OM is conductive hearing loss due to middle ear effusion. Infants with severe and ROM and persistent middle ear effusion are at risk for problems in behavior and development of speech, language, and cognitive abilities.

Selection and spread of multidrug resistant bacterial pathogens arising from extensive use of antimicrobial agents for OM is a problem for management of all diseases due to the pathogens. The careful use of strict diagnostic criteria coupled with judicious use of antibiotic therapy will direct antibiotic treatment to only those patients likely to benefit from it. Parent stress is frequent. Evidence from a large number of randomized controlled trials can help when discussing treatment options with families. Referral to an otolaryngologist should be considered if medical therapy for recurrent AOM or chronic OME (COME) has failed or been poorly tolerated, and if chronic disease or complications are present.

R. Godinho (✉)
Department of Medicine, Medical School Pontifical Catholic University of Minas Gerais, Rua Dr Chassim 208, Sete Lagoas, MG 35700-018, Brazil
e-mail: ricardogodinho@pucminas.br

T. Sih
Department of Pediatric Otolaryngology, Medical School University of São Paulo, 306 Mato Grosso St. suite 1510, São Paulo, SP 01239-040, Brazil

Global Health Disparities

OM diagnoses in children and adolescents in the USA declined by 28% between 1997 and 2007, from 345 to 247 per 1000 children younger than 18 years [4]. The youngest children (younger than 3 years) had the highest rates of OM diagnoses, and OM diagnosis rates declined by 38% from 1160 per 1000 children in 1997 to 840 in 2006 and 724 in 2007 [4]. From 1994 to 2009, the percentage of 2- to 3-year-old Canadian children with frequent OM (≥ 4 OM episodes) decreased from 26% in 1994–1995 to 12.6% in 2008–2009, a highly significant reduction ($p < 0.001$). The percentage of 2- to 3-year-old children with at least one ear infection also declined significantly over this time period from 67% in 1994–1995 to 50% in 2008–2009 ($p < 0.001$) [5].

The introduction of pneumococcal conjugate vaccines and the guidelines encouraging primary care providers to use more stringent criteria in diagnosing AOM are probably important factors in the decline in OM incidence and prevalence. The declining rates of OM have been also associated with the increase in smoke-free homes.

In contrast to the youngest children (younger than 3 years), OM diagnosis rates among children in the USA aged 3–5 years and 6–17 years increased (275–316 and 70–107, respectively) between 2006 and 2007. Males and non-Hispanic (NH) whites had higher reported OM-related physician visit rates in all age groups [6].

All children born in Southwest British Columbia, Canada, in 1999–2000 were followed until age 3 years. In this cohort of over 50,000 births, 49% had one or more OM diagnoses during the 3-year period of follow-up, whereas 8% had ROM, defined as four or more physician visits over 12 months or three or more visits during a 6-month period [7].

A prospective birth cohort study in Quebec, Canada, conducted home interviews with mothers of children from age 5 months annually until 8 years of age to determine the frequency of OM and other infections. In this cohort of 1238 families, children attending large group childcare centers had an increased OM incidence compared with those in home care before the age of

2.5 years (incidence rate ratio (IRR) = 1.62; 95% confidence interval (CI), 1.19–2.20) [8].

In 2006, the incidence rate for AOM in a study of Taiwan's pediatric population of children younger than 12 years of age was 65 cases per 1000 children [9]. The incidence density rate (IDR) per 100 child-years for ROM during a 1-year period following the baseline AOM attack was highest among children from birth to 2 years of age, with an IDR of 41.2 cases per 100 person-years, as compared with an IDR of 38.8 for 3- to 5-year-olds and an IDR of 26.7 for 6- to 12-year-olds. Boys had slightly higher IDRs than girls (34.4 vs. 32.5). The highest recurrence rates were from birth to age 2 years (40.6%) as compared with 3- to 5-year-olds (37.7%) and males (34.0%).

A cohort of all school-aged (5–14 years) Sicilian children in the primary school district of Sciacca, from September 2006 to June 2007, showed that the prevalence of OME was 6.8% for children overall and decreased with age from 12.9% in 5- to 6-year-old children to 3% among those 13–14 years old [10]. Multivariate analyses, stratified by atopy status, revealed two significant risk factors for the joint effect of atopy and OME: age (odds ratio (OR) = 2.10; CI, 1.70–2.57) and history of upper respiratory tract infection (URI; OR = 2.71; CI, 1.81–3.98).

The parents of an unselected population of 332 children at school entry (about age 5 years) in the East Berkshire district of the UK were sent postal questionnaires inquiring about various symptoms of OME, rhinitis, asthma, other atopic features, treatment for any of these problems, and possible family history of atopy [11]. About 33% had some otologic symptoms, and 6% had a high likelihood of OME. No significant correlations were found between scores of OME, eczema, urticaria, and food or drug allergies. Otologic and nasal symptoms for OME and rhinitis were highly correlated.

The prevalence of COME was 8.7% in a cohort of 1740 Turkish children aged 5–12 years. *Chronic* was defined as lasting 12 weeks (3 months) or longer [12]. Several risk factors were found to be significantly associated with COME in univariate analyses: center daycare, frequent AOM and/or URI in the past year, history of allergies, number of siblings, low level of parent's education, and maternal smoking.

The Menzies School of Health Research has been conducting ear health research in the Northern Territory of Australia since the 1980s [13–15]. The largest OM surveys involved children aged between 6 and 30 months and took place in 2001 and 2003. In this 6- to 30-month age group was found that only 10% had aerated middle ears, and 15% had chronic secretory OM. Around 20% had a perforated tympanic membrane, and another 20% had AOM without perforation. Interestingly, most of these children had asymptomatic bulging eardrums.

Indigenous children in the USA, Canada, Northern Europe, Australia, and New Zealand experience more OM than other children. In some places, indigenous children continue to suffer from the most severe forms of the disease. Higher rates of invasive pneumococcal disease, pneumonia, and chronic suppurative lung disease (including bronchiectasis) are also seen.

Conclusion

The impact of AOM on child health far exceeds the discomfort and suffering associated with individual episodes of disease. AOM is among the largest drivers of antibiotic use in children, providing support for the need of prevention of disease as an important strategy for reducing antibiotic prescribing and subsequently the emergence of resistance.

Recurrent AOM is common, with as many as 20–30% of children suffering three or more episodes before their second birthday, with potential for persistent middle ear effusion and conductive hearing loss and subsequent delay or impairment in speech and language development.

CSOM also appears to have its origins in early-onset ROM. Although now uncommon in developed countries, CSOM remains an import cause of acquired hearing loss globally, including countries such as India, Australia, and Greenland [16–20].

Finally, AOM, its treatment, and its complications impose significant economic costs on society.

Epidemiologic research continues to expand with more sophisticated research designs being implemented in diverse communities.

References

1. National Center for Health Statistics, Centers for Disease Control and Prevention, Department of Health and Human Services. Healthy People 2010: Final Review. 2011; Focus Area 28 (Objective 12):28–13. www.cdc.gov/nchs/data/hpdata2010/hp2010_final_review. Accessed Jan 2011.
2. Klein RJ, Ryskulova A, Janiszewski R, et al. Healthy people 2010, focus area 28 progress review, Round 2. Oct 2008.
3. Schappert SM, Rechtsteiner EA. Ambulatory medical care utilization estimates for 2006. Natl Health Stat Report. 2008;8:1–19.
4. Schappert SM, Rechtsteiner EA. Ambulatory medical care utilization estimates for 2007. Vital Health Stat. 13. 2011;169:1–38.
5. Thomas EM. Recent trends in upper respiratory infection, ear infection and asthma among young Canadian children. Health Rep. 2010;21:1–6.
6. Schappert SM, Rechtsteiner EA. Ambulatory medical care utilization estimates for 2006. Natl Health Stat Report. 2008;8:1–38.
7. MacIntyre EA, Karr CJ, Koehoorn M, et al. Otitis media incidence and risk factors in a population-based birth cohort. Paediatr Child Health. 2010;15:437–42.
8. Côté SM, Petitclerc A, Raynault MF, et al. Short and long-term risk of infections as a function of group child care attendance: an 8-year population-based study. Arch Pediatr Adolesc Med. 2010;164:1132–7.
9. Wang PC, Chang YH, Chuang LJ, Su HF, Li CY. Incidence and recurrence of acute otitis media in Taiwan's pediatric population. Clinics (São Paulo). 2011;66:395–9.
10. Martines F, Bentivegna D, Maira E, Sciacca V, Martines E. Risk factors for otitis media with effusion: case-control study in Sicilian schoolchildren. Int J Pediatr Otorhinolaryngol. 2011;75:754–9.
11. Umapathy D, Alles R, Scadding GK. A community based questionnaire study on the association between symptoms suggestive of otitis media with effusion, rhinitis and asthma in primary school children. Int J Pediatr Otorhinolaryngol. 2007;71:705–12
12. Gultekin E, Develioglu ON, Yener M, Ozdemir I, Kulekci M. Prevalence and risk factors for persistent otitis media with effusion in primary school children in Istanbul, Turkey. Auris Nasus Larynx. 2010;37:145–9.

13. Morris PS, Richmond P, Lehmann D, Leach AJ, Gunasekera H, Coates HL. New horizons: otitis media research in Australia. Med J Aust. 2009;191(9 Suppl):S73–7.

14. Morris PS, Leach AJ, Silberberg P, Mellon G, Wilson C, Hamilton E, et al. Otitis media in young Aboriginal children from remote communities in Northern and Central Australia: a cross-sectional survey. BMC Pediatr 2005;5:27.

15. Morris PS, Leach AJ, Halpin S, Mellon G, Gadil G, Wigger C, et al. An overview of acute otitis media in Australian Aboriginal children living in remote communities. Vaccine 2007;25(13):2389–93.

16. Jensen RG, Homoe P, Andersson M, Koch A. Long-term follow-up of chronic suppurative otitis media in a high-risk children cohort. Int J Pediatr Otorhinolaryngol. 2011;75:948–54.

17. Koch A, Homoe P, Pipper C, Hjuler T, Melbye M. Chronic suppurative otitis media in a birth cohort of children in Greenland: population-based study of incidence and risk factors. Pediatr Infect Dis J. 2011;30:25–9.

18. Leach AJ, Morris PS. The burden and outcome of respiratory tract infection in Australian and Aboriginal children. Pediatr Infect Dis J. 2007;26:S4–7.

19. Menon S, Bharadwaj R, Chowdhary A, Kaundinya DV, Palande DA. Current epidemiology of intracranial abscesses: a prospective 5 year study. J Med Microbiol. 2008;57:1259–68.

20. Morris PS, Leach AJ. Acute and chronic otitis media. Pediatr Clin North Am. 2009;56:1383–99.

Impact of Genetic Background in Otitis Media Predisposition

3

Shannon Fraser, J. Christopher Post and Margaretha L. Casselbrant

Otitis media (OM) remains one of the leading causes for pediatrician visits and antibiotic therapy in children [1]. A majority of children will suffer from at least one episode of acute otitis media (AOM) before 24 months of age [2, 3]. Complications and sequelae of OM can have disastrous consequences for children including progression to mastoiditis, labyrinthitis, cholesteatoma, hearing loss, speech delay [4], and learning disabilities. Given the prevalence of OM and the risk of devastating complications and sequelae, understanding its pathogenesis is an important public health matter.

Predisposition to the development of OM results from a complex interaction between patient and environmental factors. Well-established environmental factors that increase the risk of OM in children include daycare attendance, tobacco exposure, pacifier use, and number of siblings [2, 5]. Important patient-specific factors include male gender [2], allergy [6], and the presence of craniofacial malformations [7]. Additionally, a family history of OM is closely associated with the development of both recurrent acute otitis media (RAOM) and chronic otitis media with effusion (COME) suggesting a strong genetic component to the disease process [8].

Twin Studies

Heritability is defined as the proportion of total variance within a population that is attributable to variation in genotype [9]. Traditionally, twin studies have been used as a tool to measure the heritability of a trait within populations. Comparison of the concordance of a trait among monozygotic twins, who share identical genomes, to the concordance in dizygotic twins, sharing 50% of their genome, can provide insight into the amount of variation accounted for by genetic factors alone. Several twin studies have been conducted to investigate heritability in OM.

In a study conducted in Pittsburgh, PA, a total of 168 same-sex twin and 7 triplet sets were studied prospectively to determine the proportion of time with middle-ear effusion (MEE), episodes of MEE, and episodes of AOM. At the 2-year endpoint, the heritability for time with MEE was 73% ($p < 0.001$). The study reported discordance of 0.04 for three or more episodes of MEE in monozygotic twins compared with 0.37 for dizygotic twins ($p = 0.01$); and discordance of an episode of AOM of 0.04 in monozygotic twins

M. L. Casselbrant (✉)
Division of Pediatric Otolaryngology, Children's Hospital of Pittsburgh of UPMC, 4401 Penn Avenue, Faculty Pavillion, 7th Floor, Pittsburgh, PA 15224, USA
e-mail: casselbrantml@upmc.edu

Department of Otolaryngology, University of Pittsburgh School of Medicine, Pittsburgh, PA, USA

S. Fraser
Department of Otolaryngology, University of Pittsburgh School of Medicine, Pittsburgh, PA, USA

J. C. Post
Departments of Surgery and Microbiology, Allegheny General Hospital, Pittsburgh, PA, USA

Temple University School of Medicine and Drexel University College of Medicine, Pittsburgh, PA, USA

© Springer International Publishing Switzerland 2015

D. Preciado (ed.), *Otitis Media: State of the art concepts and treatment*, DOI 10.1007/978-3-319-17888-2_3

compared to 0.49 in dizygotic twins ($p=0.005$). The authors concluded that there was a strong genetic component to COME and AOM in the study population [10]. In a 5-year follow-up report of 83 twin sets, heritability was reported at 72% ($p<0.001$) [11]. Strengths of this study included its prospective nature, frequent otologic examinations by validated observers blinded to the patients' zygosity, and a very low drop-out rate.

The Twin Early Development Study examined all twins born in 1994 in England and Wales. This study estimated heritability of OM based on parental questionnaires for 715 sets of monozygotic twins and 658 sets of dizygotic twins. Estimated heritabilities at ages 2, 3, and 4 years were reported as 0.49, 0.66, and 0.71, respectively [12].

Linkage Analysis Studies

Encouraged by the twin studies that demonstrated a genetic component to OM, researchers have conducted several genome-wide linkage analysis studies in an effort to identify OM genetic loci that are associated with a predisposition to the development of OM. Linkage analysis takes advantage of the tendency of genetic sequences located in close proximity to each other on the same chromosome to cosegregate within a family. Genetic sequences known as markers have a known position in the genome, much like a mile marker on a highway. In linkage analysis, inheritance of the disease phenotype and various markers are compared. Markers that are close to the disease gene will tend to be inherited with the disease gene when compared to markers that are farther away from the disease gene. The likelihood for two genetic sequences to be linked is described by the logarithm of odds (LOD) score with a higher LOD indicating stronger linkage results. An LOD score of 3 is approximately equivalent to a p value of 0.0001 [13]. A major advantage of the genome-wide approach is that no a priori assumption needs to be made regarding the role of a specific gene (contrast with the candidate gene approach, see below). The genome-wide approach also provides for the discovery of novel genes. A downside of the genome-wide approach is the expense (although costs are rapidly dropping).

While there are a variety of markers used in genome studies, two will be discussed here, microsatellites and single-nucleotide polymorphisms. Microsatellites are short, repeating sequences of DNA occurring throughout the genome, although they tend to occur in noncoding DNA. A common microsatellite is known as a CA repeat and occurs every few thousand base pairs. An example would be CACACACA (i.e., four CA repeats). CA repeats can be represented as $(CA)_n$, where n is variable between alleles and may range from 2 to 100.

Microsatellites can be identified through amplification of their flanking sequences using the polymerase chain reaction (PCR). The variability of the flanking sequences allows the development of locus-specific primers. Another type of genome marker is known as a single-nucleotide polymorphism (SNP, pronounced "snip"). A SNP is a single DNA sequence variation, most commonly in the noncoding or "intron" sequences of DNA. SNPs generally are not associated with changes in phenotype.

A 2004 study conducted in Minnesota recruited families with children who had undergone tympanostomy tube placement for COME and/or recurrent otitis media (RAOM). A total of 591 individuals from 133 families were included in the analysis of 404 microsatellite markers. This group reported a statistically significant linkage of COME and/or ROM to chromosome *10q26.3* (LOD$=3.78$, $p=3.0 \times 10^{(-5)}$) and *19q13.42-q13.43* (LOD 2.61, $p=5.3 \times 10^{(-4)}$) [14]. A follow-up study reported in 2011 focused on further localizing the linkage signal previously identified on chromosome 19 [15]. Fine mapping was performed on a 5-Mb region of chromosome 19 and subsequently analyzed for marker-to-marker disequilibrium. This study confirmed the previously described linkage on chromosome 19 with a maximum LOD score of 3.75 ($p=1.6 \times 10^{(-5)}$).

A second genome-wide linkage scan reported in 2009 was performed on a cohort from Pittsburgh, PA. This study included 1506 individuals from 429 families. In the Caucasian cohort, a linkage peak at *17q12* was identified with an

LOD of 2.85. In the combined cohort of Caucasian and African-American families a peak at *10q22.3* was identified as the most significant ($p=2.6 \times 10^{(-4)}$) [16]. Interestingly, this study did not demonstrate linkage in the regions identified within the Minnesota cohort at *10q23.3* and *19q13.43*.

A genome-wide association study published in 2012 analyzed more than two million SNPs for association with OM in 416 cases and 1075 controls from the Western Australian Pregnancy Cohort Study. This study identified CAPN14 on chromosome *2p23.1* as the most highly associated with the development of OM in their population (OR1.90). The authors also noted an independent effect of an adjacent gene, GALNT12 (OR-1.60). Overall, this study reported 32 genomic regions that showed association with OM in their study population and noted that many of the top candidate genes were associated with the TGF-β pathway [17].

Candidate Gene Approach

In an effort to obviate the expense and effort of an entire genome evaluation, the candidate gene approach attempts to identify an association between the phenotype of interest and preselected genes. Generally, these genes are selected based upon a putative role in the disease in question, using current knowledge of the gene's physiological, biochemical or function, for example, selecting genes associated with the immune response when examining susceptibility to an infectious disease. While candidate gene studies are relatively inexpensive and straightforward to perform, there are several downsides to this approach: The a priori selection of candidate genes may not be correct, and novel genes will not be discovered. Candidate genes that have been considered to potentially play a role in OM susceptibility included toll-like receptors (TLRs), the TGF-β signaling pathway, surfactants, and mucins.

TLRs are known to play an important role in the activation of the innate immune system; thus, it is reasonable to assume that TLRs are good candidate genes for OM susceptibility. SNPs in TLR genes have been linked to an increased susceptibility to infections and TLR4-deficient mice have a high incidence of chronic otitis media (COM) [18].

A 2012 report by Carroll et al. compared blood samples from children with COME and RAOM ($n=70$) with those undergoing surgery for non-otologic indications ($n=70$). Reverse transcription polymerase chain reaction (RT-PCR) genotyping was performed on the blood samples for TLR2, TLR4, TLR9, and CD14. This study found no significant difference between the two groups in prevalence of SNPs within these genes [19].

A 2014 case-control study by MacArthur et al. [20]. attempted to identify candidate gene polymorphisms associated with COME. This study analyzed 170 tag-SNPs in a total of 100 case and 79 control salivary samples for association with COME. The tested genes and associated SNPs were chosen by literature review. The authors identified eight SNPs from four genes with a p value < 0.05 for association with COME. Five of the identified polymorphisms occurred in the TLR4 gene. The remaining polymorphisms occurred in the Muc5B (mucin production), SMAD2 and SMAD4 genes (TGF-β signaling pathway). Although this was a relatively small study, the authors concluded that mutations in the TLR4 gene might portend susceptibility to the development of COME [20].

The TGF-β signaling pathway has also been implicated in playing an important role in the development of OM. Multiple studies have reported association between mutations in the TGF-β1 pathway and OM. In a family-based analysis of an Australian study group, a significant association was found between severe OM and the genes FBXO11, SMAD2, and SMAD4, all known to be involved in the TGF-β1 pathway [21]. Additionally, the Minnesota COME/ROM Family Study also found an association between polymorphisms in the FBXO11 gene and the development of COME and ROM [22].

Surfactants have long been known to play an important role as tension-reducing phospholipoprotein in the lung. Surfactants are also expressed in the middle ear, and more recently research has recognized their role in innate immunity, specifically opsonisation [23]. Studies to further investigate the role of surfactant in the development of OM have been somewhat inconclusive. A study of Finnish children published in 2001 reported that a specific haplotype ($6A^4$–$1A^5$) of surfactant A had a higher incidence in patients with RAOM compared to a control group [24]. A subsequent study investigated the same haplotype in a group of children from Connecticut. Contrary to the Finnish study, this report found a protective association of the $6A^4$–$1A^5$ haplotype with OM [25].

Mucins are glycosylated proteins that play an integral role in the mucociliary transport system that functions to maintain ventilation of the middle ear [26]. The finding that mucins are overproduced in the middle ear in cases of chronic OM [27] led to further investigation of mucin gene polymorphisms in OM patients. A 2010 study by Ubell et al. found an association between the MUC5AC-b allele and the development of OM in their case-control study of 60 patients [28]. In the Minnesota family cohort there was a significant association between SNPs in the region of MUC5AC/MUC5B and MUC2 and the development of OM. However, only the MUC2 association could be confirmed in their replication study [29].

Human studies have also supported the role of FBXO11 as a potential susceptibility gene for the development of OM. An Australian study group demonstrated an association between SNPs within the FBXO11 gene and the development of OM in their study, which included 561 individuals from 434 families [21]. Similarly, a univariate genetic analysis performed on the Minnesota COME/ROM Family Study (142 families, 619 individuals) demonstrated evidence of an association between rs2134056, an SNP within the FBXO11 gene, and the development of COME/ROM ($p = 0.02$) [22].

In addition to the abovementioned candidate genes, there are studies investigating the role of numerous other components of the immune system and their association with OM. Various cytokines, including IL6 [30], IL10 [31], and IL1 [32] have all been implicated in the pathogenesis of OM; however, many of these studies have failed to be replicated.

Animal Models

Animal models have played an important role in the investigation of many human diseases. Several murine models for OM have been developed namely the Jeff, Junbo, and C3H/HeJ lines.

The Jeff *(Jf)* mouse carries a single-point mutation in the FBXO11 gene, rendering it nonfunctional. This mouse line develops spontaneous chronic OM [33]. Mice heterozygous for the Jeff mutation will develop COME even if raised in pathogen-free conditions [34], suggesting an anatomic rather than immune deficiency contributing to ear disease in this line. These mice have craniofacial abnormalities including a shortened snout and a narrow, bent Eustachian tube [35].

Similarly, the Junbo *(Jbo)* mouse develops spontaneous COME in the perinatal period due to a loss of function in the gene Evi1 [36]. Although the Jbo mouse displays no craniofacial abnormalities, heterozygotes develop OM even in pathogen-free conditions. Both FBXO11 and Evi1 proteins are known to interact with the TGF-β signaling pathway [35, 37]. Although not fully understood, one proposed mechanism by which the Evi1 mutation potentially contributes to the development of OM is through upregulation of mucin transcription leading to the enhancement of effusive processes in the middle ear.

The C3H/HeJ mouse model has a single mutation within the TLR4 gene and is associated with a 50 % incidence of COME by 8 months of age. This mouse demonstrates no craniofacial abnormalities, and its predisposition to OM is proposed to be a result of deficient response to the lipopolysaccharide of gram-negative bacteria [18].

Recently, a novel mouse model has been developed that has a predisposition to the development of spontaneous MEE. This mouse has a specific mutation in a G protein couple receptor (GPCR) encoded by the Oxgr1 gene. 82 % of mice with an Oxgr1 knockout developed middle-ear inflammation with hearing loss. Histological evaluation demonstrated inflammatory cells, changes in the mucosal epithelium and MEE, making this knockout an excellent model to examine mucin regulation in MEE [38].

Otitis Media has a clear and well-documented tendency to run in families, and a significant body of literature exists investigating the genetic basis for OM. Heritability studies provide strong evidence for a genetic component in both COME and RAOM. Numerous studies have demonstrated associations between specific genes and risk for the development of OM; unfortunately, many of these studies report conflicting findings. Polymorphisms of various cytokines have been shown to increase the risk of developing OM in study populations; however, most of these associations have not been reproduced by subsequent studies.

The development of OM involves a complex interaction between a patient's environment and their unique genetic makeup. Elucidating the specifics of the genes responsible for predisposition of OM is a challenging problem due to this complexity. Genetics appear to be important to the development of OM on various levels including contributions to structural and anatomical factors as well as to variations in immune function.

References

1. Freid VM, Makuc DM, Rooks RN. Ambulatory health care visits by children: principal diagnosis and place of visit. Vital Health Stat. 1998;13(137):1–23.
2. Paradise JL, Rockette E, Colborn DK, et al. Otitis media in 2253 Pittsburgh-area infants: prevalence and risk factors during the first two years of life. Pediatrics. 1997;99:318–33.
3. Daly KA, Hoffman HJ, Kvaerner KJ, et al. Epidemiology, natural history and risk factors: panel report from the Ninth International Research Conference on Otitis Media. Int J Pediatr Otorhinolaryngol. 2010;74:231–40.
4. Goldstein NA, Casselbrant ML, Bluestone CD, Kurs-Lasky M. Intratemporal complications of acute otitis media in infants and children. Otolaryngol Head Neck Surg. 1998;119(5):444–54.
5. Lubianca Neto JF, Hemb L, Silva DB. Systematic literature review of modifiable risk factors for recurrent acute otitis media in childhood. J Pediatr (Rio J). 2006;82:87–96.
6. Chantzi FM, Kafetzis DA, Bairamis T, et al. IgE sensitization, respiratory allergy symptoms, and heritability independently increase the risk of otitis media with effusion. Allergy. 2006;61:332–6.
7. Di Francesco R, Paulucci B, Nery C, Bento RF. Craniofacial morphology and otitis media with effusion in children. Int J Pediatr Otorhinolaryngol. 2008;72(8):1151–8.
8. Daly KA, Rich SS, Levine S, et al. The family study of otitis media: design and disease and risk factor profiles. Genet Epidemiol. 1996;13:451–68.
9. Visscher PM, Hill WG, Wray NR. Heritability in the genomics era—concepts and misconceptions. Nat Rev Genet. 2008;9:255–66.
10. Casselbrant ML, Mandel EM, Fall PA, et al. The heritability of otitis media: a twin and triplet study. JAMA. 1999;282:2125–30.
11. Casselbrant ML, Mandel EM, Rockette HE, et al. The genetic component of middle ear disease in the first 5 years of life. Arch Otolaryngol Head Neck Surg. 2004;130:273–8.
12. Rovers M, Haggard M, Gannon M, et al. Heritability of symptom domains in otitis media: a longitudinal study of 1373 twin pairs. Am J Epidemiol. 2002;155:958–64.
13. Dawn Teare M, Berrett JH. Genetic linkage studies. Lancet. 2005;366:1036–44.
14. Daly KA, Brown WM, Segade F, et al. Chronic and recurrent otitis media: a genome scan for susceptibility loci. Am J Hum Genet. 2004;75:988–97.
15. Chen WM, Allen EK, Mychaleckyj JC, Chen F, Hou X, Rich SS, Daly KA, Sale MM. Significant linkage at chromosome 19q for otitis media with effusion and/or recurrent otitis media (COME/ROM). BMC Med Genet. 2011;12:124. doi:10.1186/1471-2350-12-124.
16. Casselbrant ML, Mandel EM, Jung J, et al. Otitis media: a genome-wide linkage scan with evidence of susceptibility loci within the 17q12 and 10q22.3 regions. BMC Med Genet. 2009;10:85.
17. Rye MS, Warrington NM, Scaman ES, Vijayasekaran S, Coates HL, Anderson D, Pennell CE, Backwell JM, Jamieson SE. Genome-wide association study to identify the genetic determinants of otits media susceptibility in childhood. PLoS ONE. 2012;7(10):e48215.
18. Macarthur CJ, Hefeneider SH, Kempton B, Trune BR. C3H/HeJ Mouse model for spontaneous chronic otitis media. Laryngoscope. 2006;116:1071–9.
19. Carroll SR, Zald PB, Soler ZM, Milczuk HA, Trune DR, MacArthur CJ. Innate immunity gene single nucleotide polymorphisms and otitis media. Int J Pediatr Otorhinolaryngol. 2012;76:976–9.
20. Macarthur CJ, Wilmot B, Wang L, Schuller M, Lightall J, Trune D. Genetic susceptibility to chronic otitis media with effusion: *Candidate* gene single nucleotide polymorphisms. Laryngoscope. 2014;124(5):1229–35.

21. Rye MS, et al. FBXO11, a regulator of the TGFβ pathway, is associated with severe otitis media in Western Australian children. Genes Immun. 2011;12(5):352–9.

22. Segade F, et al. Association of the FBXO11 gene with chronic otitis media with effusion and recurrent otitis media: the Minnesota COME/ROM Family Study. Arch Otolaryngol Head Neck Surg. 2006;132(7):729–33.

23. Wright JR. Immunoregulatory functions of surfactant proteins. Nat Rev Immunol. 2005;5:58–68.

24. Ramet M, Lofgren J, Alho OP, et al. Surfactant protein-A gene locus associated with recurrent otitis media. J Pediatr. 2001;138:266–8.

25. Pettigrew M, Gent JF, Zhu Y, et al. Association of surfactant protein A polymorphisms with otitis media in infants at risk for asthma. BMC Med Genet. 2006;7:68.

26. Lin J, Tsuprun V, Kawano H, et al. Characterization of mucins in human middle ear and Eustachian tube. Am J Phsiol Lung Cell Mol Physiol. 2001;280:L1157–67.

27. Preciado D, Goyal S, Rahimi M, et al. MUC5B is the predominant mucin glycoprotein in chronic otitis media fluid. Pediatr Res. 2010;68:231–6.

28. Ubell ML, Khampang P, Kerschner JE. Mucin gene polymorphisms in otitis media patients. Laryngoscope. 2010;120:132–8.

29. Sale MM, Chen WM, Weeks DE, et al. Evaluation of 15 functional candidate genes for association with chronic otitis media with effusion and/or recurrent otitis media (COME/ROM). PLoS ONE. 2011;6(8):e22297.

30. Patel JA, Nair S, Revai K, et al. Association of proinflammatory cytokine gene polymorphisms with susceptibility to otitis media. Pediatrics. 2006;118:2273–9.

31. Emonts M, Veenhoven RH, Wiertsema SP, et al. Genetic polymorphisms in immunoresponse genes THFA, IL6, IL10 and TLR4 are associated with recurrent acute otitis media. Pediatrics. 2007;120:814–23.

32. Joki-Erkkila VP, Puhakka H, Hurme M. Cytokine gene polymorphism in recurrent acute otitis media. Arch Otolaryngol Head Neck Surg. 2002;128:17–20.

33. Haridsty-Hughes RE, et al. A mutation in the F-box gene, Fbxo11, causes otitis media in the Jeff mouse. Hum Mol Genet. 2006;15(22):3273–9.

34. Rye MS, Bhutta MF, Cheeseman MT, et al. Unraveling the genetics of otitis media: from mouse to human and back again. Mamm Genome. 2011;22:66–82.

35. Hardisty RE, Erven A, Logan K, Morse S, Guionaud S, et al. The deaf mouse mutant Jeff (Jf) is a single gene model of otitis media. J Assoc Res Otolaryngol. 2003;4:130–8.

36. Parkinson N, et al. Mutation at the Evi1 locus in Junbo mice causes susceptibility to otitis media. PLoS Genet. 2006;2(10):e149.

37. Tateossian H, et al. Regulation of TGF-beta signalling by Fbxo11, the gene mutated in the Jeff otitis media mouse mutant. Pathogenetics. 2009;2(1):5.

38. Kerschner JE, Hong W, Taylor SR, Kerschner JA, Khampang P, Wrege KC, North PE. A novel model of spontaneous otitis media with effusion (OME) in the Oxgr1 knock-out mouse. Int J Pediatr Otorhinolaryngol. 2013;77(1):79–84.

Risk Factors for Recurrent Acute Otitis Media and Chronic Otitis Media with Effusion in Childhood

José Faibes Lubianca Neto and Tania Sih

Host-associated Risk Factors for RAOM

Allergy

Although there is epidemiologic, mechanical, and therapeutic evidence showing that allergic rhinitis contributes to the pathogenesis of otitis media, there are still many controversies about its influence as a risk factor. Kraemer et al. [1], in a case-control study, compared the prevalence of atopic symptoms in 76 cases submitted to tympanotomy for the placement of ventilation tubes with 76 controls paired by age, sex, and season of the year on admission to have general pediatric surgery performed. The cases presented with approximately four times more complaints of atopic symptoms. Through a cohort of 707 children with recurrent acute otitis media (RAOM), Pukander and Karma [2] found more persistent

J. F. L. Neto (✉)
Department of Otolaryngology and Pediatric Otorhinolaryngology, Santo Antônio Children's Hospital, Rua Dona Laura, 320/9th floor, Porto Alegre, RS 90430-090, Brazil
e-mail: Lubianca@otorrinospoa.com.br

Department of Clinical Surgery, Medical School of Federal University of Health Sciences, Porto Alegre, RS, Brazil

T. Sih
Department of Pediatric Otolaryngology, Medical School University of São Paulo, 306 Mato Grosso St. suite 1510, São Paulo, SP 01239-040, Brazil
e-mail: tsih@amcham.com.br

middle-ear effusion (MEE) for 2 months or longer in children with atopic manifestations than in those that were non-allergic. Bernstein et al. [3] followed up 77 children who had RAOM with chronic MEE, and who had at least one ventilation tube placement performed. There was increased IgE in the MEE in 14 out of 32 children with allergic rhinitis, compared with 2 out of 45 children considered to be nonallergic. In an interesting German cohort study through the first two years of life, children diagnosed with otitis media during infancy were at greater risk for developing late-onset allergic eczema and asthma during school age, and associations were stronger for frequent otitis media [4].

On the other hand, there are also well-delineated articles on allergic rhinitis, which have not been able to demonstrate association with RAOM [5–7]. Interestingly, contributing to this discordance, there are two meta-analyses of risk factors for RAOM with conflicting results. Whereas Uhary et al. [8] did not find significance of the association of atopy and RAOM, Zhang et al. [9] have shown a significant pooled odds ratio of 1.36 (confidence interval, CI 1.13–1.64).

Craniofacial Abnormalities

There is higher incidence of otitis media in children with uncorrected cleft palate than in normal children, mainly when considering those aged up to 2 years [10]. When, however, the cleft is corrected, RAOM is reduced [11], possibly because it allows improved Eustachian tube function [12]. In a retrospective cohort, Boston et al. [13] demonstrated that the presence of craniofacial deformities increased the chance of the child requiring multiple interventions for ventilation tube placements. Otitis media is also more prevalent in children with craniofacial abnormalities and Down's syndrome.

Gastroesophageal Reflux (GER)

Much of the evidence about the association of Gastroesophageal reflux (GER) and RAOM is of level III or IV, and comes from reports on cases or series of patients and from studies in animals. In 2001, four cases were reported of adults with chronic otitis media that was difficult to resolve and who, after diagnosis of GER, had been confirmed by pHmetry and endoscopy, started treatment with omeprazole and had their conditions resolved. One of these patients restarted bilateral otorrhea after suspension of the drug and had the situation controlled again with the reintroduction of omeprazole [14].

After 2002, several studies were carried out. A randomized clinical trial in rats showed that infusion of hydrochloric acid/pepsin solution in the rhinopharynx was capable of causing dysfunction in the pressure regulation and mucocilliary depuration of the middle ear, contrasting to the effects of a saline infusion in the region [15]. Rosmanic et al. [16], by means of pHmetry, demonstrated pathologic GER in 55.6% of children with RAOM or chronic suppurative otitis media (COME), and as a result recommended double channel pHmetry in children who did not respond to conventional otitis media treatments. Tasker et al. [17] measured the pepsin concentration in MEE samples, and showed that 83% of them contained pepsin/pepsinogen at a concentration over 1000 times higher in relation to the serum concentration, concluding that gastric juice reflux may be the major cause of MEE in children. The same group of authors in a more sophisticated study reproduced their previous results and concluded that "it is almost certain that pepsin in MEE comes from acid content re-

flux and that there may therefore, be a role for anti-reflux therapy in the treatment of COME" [18]. This enthusiasm was not confirmed in the conclusions of other publications, as the study of Antonelli et al. [19], for example, who measured the total pepsinogen concentration in 26 acute otorrhea samples after ventilation tube placement and found pepsinogen in some cases, but at low concentrations, lower than normal serum levels. By other means, Pitkaranta et al. [20] also did not find evidence of the association of MEE and GER. Analyzing the presence of *Helicobacter pylori* through serological tests to detect antigens and through adenoids and MEE cultures, they found only 20% of the serological tests positive, and in none of the cases was there growth of the germ in adenoid or middle-ear cultures.

In a recent systematic review dealing only with the association between otitis media and gastroesophageal reflux, Miura et al. [21] concluded that "the prevalence of GER in children with COME/RAOM may be higher than the overall prevalence for children. Presence of pepsin/pepsinogen in MEE could be related to physiologic reflux. A cause-effect relationship between pepsin/pepsinogen in MEE and otitis media is unclear. Anti-reflux therapy of otitis media cannot be endorsed based on the existing research."

Adenoids

Those that defend the association between adenoid tissue hyperplasia and RAOM or COME base it on three different types of evidence. There are those that prefer articles pointing out great correlation (approximately 70%) between the rhinopharyngeal bacteria and those cultivated in the MEE in acute episodes [22] or those that point towards a larger number of colony counts in adenoid cultures coming from cases operated on for RAOM as compared with those operated on for obstruction [23]. The theory that adenoids functioning as a bacterial reservoir is more accepted currently than the theory of mechanical obstruction of the tube by adenoidal growth, a fact rarely proved in clinical practice [23]. Notably, randomized clinical trials have demonstrated a positive effect of adenoidectomy on reducing various end points related to otitis media [24–27].

However, there are well-delineated and well-conducted randomized clinical trials with conflicting results, demonstrating that adenoidectomy alone or associated with ventilation tube placement does not play a role in the prophylaxis of RAOM in children younger than 2 years [28, 29] at least at the first ventilation tube placement [27].

A recent meta-analysis of risk factors for RAOM [9] analyzed the potential role of large adenoids as a risk factor for RAOM. The meta-analysis examined two factors that may be linked to the presence of large adenoids-chronic nasal obstruction and snoring. Whereas results did not show any association of chronic nasal obstruction with RAOM, it showed that persistent snoring almost doubled the frequency of RAOM (OR 1.96; CI 1.78–2.16).

In conclusion, it would appear that original investigations dealing with adenoid hyperplasia and risk of RAOM or COME are lacking, and that the level of existing evidence is primarily based on expert opinion (level of evidence V) or indirect end points. The evidence comes from studies that assess the effect of adenoidectomy on events related to otitis media. It would seem that adenoidectomy is more efficient in the treatment of COME than in RAOM, and the majority of authors agree that adenoidectomy must be performed, irrespective of the size of the adenoids [30], at least when the second ventilation tube placement is performed (level of evidence I).

Genetic Susceptibility

There is anatomic, physiologic, and epidemiologic evidence showing a genetic predisposition to RAOM. In a huge prevalence study in Greenland, the positive parental history for RAOM was one of the two factors that remained a significant predictor of RAOM after the logistic regression was performed [31]. In the meta-analysis of Uhari et al. [8], positive history of acute otitis media (AOM) in any other member of the family, increased the risk for AOM in a child by 2.63 times (CI 1.86–3.72). A marker of genetic inheritance, the HLA-A2 antigen, was found more frequently and the HLA-A3 less frequently in children with RAOM than in healthy children [32, 33].

The strongest evidence of a genetic susceptibility to RAOM was shown in studies evolving twins and triplets. There are two retrospective studies. The first one, with 2750 Norwegian twin pairs, has estimated the heritability in 74% in girls and 45% in boys [34]. In the second study, with a sample of 1373 twin pairs, the estimated heritability in the ages of 2, 3, and 4 years to RAOM was, in the average, 0.57 [35]. In the prospective twins and triplets Pittsburgh study, where monthly monitoring of the middle ear was done, the estimated heritability of otitis media at the 2-year end point was 0.79 in girls and 0.64 in boys [36]. Of the original 140 pairs of twins and triplets with determined zigosity, 114 were followed up to the age of 3 and the 83 pairs followed up to the age of 5. The correlation between twins for the proportion of time with MEE was significantly higher in the monozygotic (0.65–0.77) than in the dizygotic (0.31–0.39) twins for each year until the third year. Later, it decreased, a result explained by the decrease in the incidence of otitis media in the older children. The estimates of discordance for three or more episodes of MEE in monozygotic and dizygotic twins followed up to the 5 years was 0.02 and 0.40, respectively (p =0.07). The estimated heritability of the proportion of time with MEE in the first 5 years of life was 72% (p <0.001). The correspondent estimative for boys and girls separately was 0.66 and 0.75, respectively. The results of the 5-year study still continue to support a strong genetic component to otitis media [37].

Another approach to get clues to the genetic susceptibility to RAOM is the linkage studies searching for candidates genes that predisposes to RAOM in the whole genome. As otitis media is a multifactorial disease in humans, it is not probable that one unique gene is the cause of otitis media. Linkage studies have already shown that there are some hotspots in the genome for RAOM. The first linkage study was performed by Daly et al. [38] that provided evidence of linkage of COME and RAOM to 10q26.3 and to 19q13.43. Another study was conducted at

Pittsburgh on a population of full siblings, two or more, who had a history of tympanostomy tube insertion due to a significant history of otitis media, their parent(s) and other full sibling(s) with no history of tympanostomy tube insertion. The study did not provide evidence for linkage in the previously reported regions. Most significant linkage peak was on chromosome 17q12, that include AP2B1, CCL5, and a cluster of other CCl genes, and in 10q22.3, STFPA2 [39].

The genetic predisposition to otitis media is only starting to be discovered. Potential therapeutic targets are the genes regulating mucin expression, mucus production, and host response to bacteria in the middle ear (Li et al. 2013). The identification of the susceptibility genes to otitis media could improve the knowledge of the otitis media physiopathology and provide development of molecular diagnostic methods that could be used to establish the risk for otitis media of a specific child and perhaps modify the follow-up and the treatment according to this established risk.

Environmental Risk Factors for RAOM

Upper Respiratory Tract Infections (URTI)

Both epidemiologic evidence and clinical experience strongly suggest that otitis media is frequently a complication of URTI. The incidence of COME is greater during autumn and winter months, and less in summer in both hemispheres [40, 41], parallel to the incidence of AOM [42, 43], and URTI [40, 41]. URTI increases the incidence of AOM. In a meta-analysis by Zhang et al. [9], pooled analyses showed that URTI increase the risk of otitis media almost sevenfold (OR 6.59; 95% CI 3.13–13.89). Revai et al. [44] evaluated 623 URTI episodes in 112 children (6–35 months of age) and found an AOM associated incidence of 30%. In another prospective cohort [4] of 294 healthy children (6 month to 3 years of age), the overall incidence of OM complicating URTI was 61%, including 37% AOM and 24% COME. Having had recurrent URTI in

the past 12 months was one of the variables in the multivariable model that increased the risk of RAOM in a 2010 study [45]. This evidence supports the assumption that URTI plays an important role in the etiology of otitis media (level of evidence II), and prevention of viruses may decrease the incidence of RAOM.

Studies that have tried to isolate MEE virus in children have indeed demonstrated both viral antigens and even live viruses in MEE [46–48]. Among the various mechanisms by which URTI may predispose patients to RAOM and COME, are inflammation and harm to the mucocilliary movement of the epithelium that lines the auditory tube, which has been demonstrated both experimentally [49] and clinically [50]. Viral URTI promotes the replication of the bacterial infection and increases inflammation in the nasopharynx and ET.

Day-care Center Attendance

Day-care center attendance has been considered a major risk factor for developing RAOM for a long time. Alho et al. [51] examined questionnaires that were sent to 2512 randomly selected Finnish children's parents and also reviewed their clinical record cards and found an estimated relative risk of 2.06 (95% CI 1.81–2.34) for development of AOM in children that frequented day-care centers when compared with care in their own homes. It was also demonstrated that children in day-care centers are more prone to needing ventilation tube insertion than children cared for at home. In another analysis, the risk found for COME was 2.56 (95% CI 1.17–5.57) [52].

It would appear that the setting of where the child is cared for influences this association. It has been shown that susceptibility to AOM diminished in a group of children who are cared for in family homes, in comparison with day-care center attendance [5, 6]. The prevalence of negative pressure in the middle ear and type B tympanograms, indicative of MEE, are greater in children cared for in day-care centers with many others; intermediate in children cared for in family homes with fewer "companions" and less still in children cared for at home [52, 53]. In the meta-analysis of Uhari et al. [8], the risk of AOM also increased with child care outside the home (RR 2.45; 95% CI 1.51–3.98) and although on a lower scale, also with care in family homes (RR 1.59; 95% CI 1.19–2.13). It is postulated that the risk is proportional to the number of "companions" the children are in contact with [5, 6]. Large group child care centers increase otitis media incidence and were defined as those in which professional educators provided care for up to 10 groups of 8–12 children in the same setting [54]. A possible mechanism is related to the greater number of URTI presented by children that are exposed to many other children [55]. In conclusion, there would appear that there is little doubt here, day-care center attendance is a risk factor for RAOM and COME (level of evidence II). Alho et al. [56] in a hypothetical cohort estimated that if 825 children were transferred from day-care centers to home care and followed up for 2 years, approximately two out of five affected would escape RAOM.

Family Size (Siblings)

Greater incidence of AOM and COME is described in children belonging to big families (especially if many of them are under 5 years of age) [10, 57]. History of RAOM in siblings is considered to be a risk factor [5, 58]. Birth order was also associated with the rate of otitis media episodes and with the percentage of time with MEE, with the first child having the lower rates in the first 2 years of life than the others with older siblings [58]. The chance of RAOM increases 4.18 times (95% CI 2.74–6.36) in the younger generation among siblings [59]. Also, having more than one sibling was found to be significantly related to early onset of otitis media [60].

The findings of the studies dealing with this risk factor, however, are not unanimous. A population study by Vinther et al. [61] did not demonstrate that family size was a risk factor for otitis media. The same was seen in the classical cohort study by Teele et al. [62]. It is very difficult to

separate the influence of genetics from care in day-care centers and the socioeconomic level itself (families with lower purchasing power tend to be larger) from the exclusive effect of the number of siblings as a risk factor. In the meta-analysis of Uhari et al. [8], which pooled the results of two previous conflicting studies [5, 62], an increase of 92% in the incidence of otitis media if there is at least one sibling was shown (RR 1.92; 95% CI 1.29–2.85).

Passive Smoking

It is one of the most studied risk factors for RAOM. From 1978 to 1985, only case-control and cross-sectional studies with some methodological limitations were published, followed by well-designed cohorts later in 1985 and meta-analysis in 1996. The first class of studies were more controversial, showing positive [1, 63–65] and negative [61, 66–69] associations between otitis media (AOM, COME) and second-hand smoke exposure.

The first prospective cohort study of Iversen et al. [70] studying 337 children recruited in day-care centers, showed smoking as a risk for COME, with the additional finding that the risk associated with passive smoking increased with age. Zielhius et al. [70] followed up a cohort of 1463 children and found a relative risk for COME of 1.07 (95% CI 0.90–1.26) in children exposed to passive smoking. In 1993, follow up of 698 children demonstrated that the presence of smokers and greater numbers of cigarette packs smoked daily in the house increased time with MEE [71]. Ey et al. [72] prospectively analyzed 1013 children from birth to 1 year old, demonstrating that mothers' heavy smoking (20 or more cigarettes/day) was a significant risk factor for RAOM, with a relative risk of 1.78 (95% CI 1.01–3.11) in multivariate analysis. In another prospective cohort involving 918 children, it was demonstrated that children whose mothers smoked 20 or more cigarettes a day were at significantly increased risk of having four or more episodes of AOM (RR 1.8; 95% CI 1.1–3.0) and of having the first episode of AOM much earlier (RR 1.3;

95% CI 1.0–1.8). The risk of RAOM increased parallel to the number of cigarettes smoked [73]. In another prospective cohort study, children who underwent insertion of tympanostomy tubes were followed up for 12 months. Maternal smoking increased the risk for RAOM (OR 4.15; CI 1.45–11.9) after insertion of ventilation tubes [74].

There are at least four studies that measured objectively the exposure to tobacco smoking through a nicotine metabolite (cotinine) in saliva and urine. In 1987, Etzel [75] conducted a retrospective cohort of 9 years with 132 day-care children. He measured exposure to passive smoking through salivary cotinine concentration. The incidence density rate of MEE was 1.39 (95% CI 1.15–1.69) and 1.38 (95% CI 1.21–1.56) in the first year and in the first 3 years of life, respectively. However, the significance disappeared with the introduction of other variables in the logistic regression. In 1989, Strachan et al. [66] did not find association between salivary cotinine and otitis media. In 1999, Daly et al. [6] were unable to demonstrate association between the early onset of AOM and the rate of cotinine–creatinine in urine. In 2001, Ilicali et al. [76] found that around 74% of the children in the "case" group required surgical intervention by RAOM or COME and 55% in the "control" group were exposed to passive smoking ($p = 0.046$).

At least three meta-analyses studied the association of passive smoking with RAOM and COME. The first was done by Uhari et al. [8], demonstrating a significant increase of 66% (RR 1.66; 95% CI 1.33–2.06). Strachan and Cook [63] demonstrated estimated relative risks, if at least one of the parents smoked, of 1.48 (95% CI 1.08–2.04) for RAOM, of 1.38 (95% CI 1.23–1.55) for MEE, and of 1.21 (95% CI 0.95–1.53) for COME. Finally, Zhang et al. [9] calculated a risk of 1.92 (95% CI 1.29–2.85) for RAOM.

In conclusion, although some authors have declared the relationship between RAOM and COME with passive smoking as firm [77], others are against such affirmation [78]. It may be said that passive smoking does not increase the chance of nonrecurrent AOM (level of evidence IV). With regard to RAOM and COME, passive smoking is a probable risk factor (level of evidence II).

Breast-feeding

The majority of researchers believe that breast-feeding protects against otitis media. In a prospective cohort of Saarinen et al. [78], children that were breast-fed up to 6 months of age did not have any episodes of AOM, whereas 10% of those that started with cows' milk before they were 2 months old presented with such episodes in this period. At the end of the first year, the incidence of two or more episodes of otitis was 6% in the first and 19% in the second group. From the end of the first up to the third year, four or more episodes of otitis occurred in 6% of breast-fed children, compared with 26% of those artificially fed. Although there were many subjects lost to follow-up in the study, it was shown that prolonged breast-feeding (6 months or longer) protects the child against RAOM up to the third year of life. The group that used cows' milk had the first AOM episode much earlier.

The retrospective study of Cunningham et al. comprising 503 patients, found 3.7 and 9.1 episodes per 1000 patients/week for the breast-fed and artificially fed groups, respectively. In this study, with adequate control of confounding factors, significant difference was shown (total number of episodes—23 vs. 182) [79]. Case-control studies also showed a significantly lower number of episodes of otitis in the first 2 years in breast-fed children in comparison with those that were fed with cows' milk (0.3 episodes (9/30) compared with the 2.9 (86/30) episodes) [80]. Stahlberg et al. [7], in a case-control study with 115 children "prone to otitis," hospitalized to have adenoidectomy performed, demonstrated association between the duration of breast-feeding and age of introduction to cows' milk with RAOM. Duncan et al. [81] followed up 1013 nursing infants for 1 year and demonstrated that those that were exclusively breast-fed for 4 months or longer, had half the number of AOM episodes, compared with non-breast-fed infants, and 50% less otitis than those that were breast-fed for less than 4 months. A cohort of 306 children followed up for the first 2 years demonstrated that between 6 and 12 months of age, the cumulative incidence of first episodes increased from

25 to 51 % in exclusively breast-fed infants and from 54 to 76 % in nursing infants fed on formulas since birth. The peak of AOM incidence and MEE was inversely related to the breast-feeding rates beyond 3 months of age. There was double the risk for the first episode of AOM in nursing infants exclusively fed on formulas, compared with nursing infants exclusively breast-fed for 6 months during the same period of life [82]. Mandel et al. [83] followed up 148 children, aged 1.0–8.6 years, and showed that the lack of breast-feeding was one of the significant predictors of otitis media with effusion (OME) and AOM incidence. However, there are some studies that have not found a protective effect of breast-feeding in the risk of otitis media [84, 85].

One of the mechanisms involved in the association between breast-feeding and otitis media is "positional otitis media," according to which, children breast-fed in a unsuitable position (lying down) are at greater risk for otitis media [81, 86]. A cohort with 698 children followed up from birth to 2 years of age demonstrated that the supine breast-feeding position was associated with earlier onset of COME [71].

In conclusion, the majority of the studies, corroborated by findings of meta-analysis showing that children breast-fed for at least 3 months reduced the risk of AOM by 13 % (RR 0.87; 95 % CI 0.79–0.95) by Uhari et al. [8], demonstrated that breast-feeding has a protective effect against middle-ear disease (level of evidence II). However, there is controversy with respect to the optimal duration of breast-feeding required for protection. A study that focused on the duration of the protection given by breast-feeding after it ceases demonstrated that the risk of AOM is significantly reduced for up to 4 months after it stops. Approximately 12 months after breast-feeding has stopped, the risk is virtually the same among those that were or were not breast-fed [87].

Use of Pacifier

Niemela et al. [88], in a sample of 938 children, demonstrated that those that used pacifiers had a greater risk of presenting with RAOM than those who did not use them. Following 845 day-care children prospectively, Niemela et al. [89, 90] found that the use of a pacifier increased the annual incidence of AOM and was responsible for up to 25 % of the episodes of the disease. Warren et al. [91] demonstrated that pacifier sucking was significantly associated with otitis media from the 6th to the 9th month and presented a strong trend towards statistical significance in the period from 9 to 12 months ($p = 0.56$). Lastly, in the meta-analysis of Uhari et al. [8], the use of a pacifier increased the risk for AOM by 25 % (estimated RR 1.24; 95 % CI 1.06–1.46) (level of evidence II).

Through an open randomized clinical trial, 14 baby welfare clinics were paired in accordance with the number of children and social class of the parents they served. One clinic in each pair was randomly allocated for intervention, while the other served as control. Intervention consisted of a leaflet explaining the deleterious effects of pacifier use and gave instructions for restricting it (basically to use the pacifier only at the time of going to sleep). A total of 272 children under 18 months of age were recruited from the intervention clinics and 212 from control clinics. After intervention, there was a 21 % decrease in continuous pacifier use from 7 to 18 months of age ($p = 0.0001$), and the occurrence of AOM was 29 % lower among children from the intervention clinics. The children that did not use the pacifier continually in any of the clinics had 33 % fewer episodes of AOM than the children that used them.

References

1. Kraemer JK, Richardson MA, Weis NS, Furukawa CT, Shapiro GG, Pierson WE, et al. Risk factors for persistent middle-ear effusions. JAMA. 1983;249:1022–5.
2. Pukander J, Karma P. Persistence of middle-ear effusion and its risk factors after an acute attack of otitis media with effusion. In: Lim DJ, Bluestone CD, Klein JO, Nelson JD, editors. Recent advances in otitis media. Proceedings of the fourth international symposium. Toronto: BC Decker; 1988, p. 8–11.
3. Bernstein JM, Lee J, Conboy K, Ellis E, Li P. The role of IgE mediated hypersensitivity in recurrent otitis media with effusion. Am J Otol. 1983;5:66–9.

4. MacIntyre EA, Karr CJ, Koehoorn M, et al. Otitis media incidence and risk factors in a population-based birth cohort. Paediatr Child Health. 2010;15:437–42.
5. Pukander J, Luotonem J, Timonen M, Karma P. Risk factors affecting the occurrence of acute otitis media among 2-3 year-old urban children. Acta Otolaryngol. 1985;100:260–5.
6. Stahlberg MR. The influence of form of day-care in occurrence of upper respiratory tract infections among young children. Acta Pediatr Scand. 1980;282:1–87.
7. Stahlberg MR, Ruskanen O, Virolainen E. Risk factors for recurrent otitis media. Pediatr Infect Dis. 1986;5:30–2.
8. Uhari M, Matsyaari K, Niemela M. A meta-analytic review of the risk factor for acute otitis media. Clin Infect Dis. 1996;22:1079–83.
9. Zhang Y, Xu M, Zhang J, Zeng L, Wang Y, Zheng KY. Risk factors for chronic and recurrent otitis media. A meta-analysis. PloS ONE. 2014;9:e86397.
10. Bluestone CD. Studies in otitis media: Children's Hospital of Pittsburgh—University of Pittsburgh Progress Report—2004. Laryngoscope. 2004;114(Suppl 105):1–26.
11. Frable MA, Brandon GT. Theogaraj SD. Velar closure and ear tubings as a primary procedure in the repair of cleft palates. Laryngoscope. 1985;95:1044–6.
12. Doyle WJ, Reilly JS, Jardini L, Rovnak S. Effect of palatoplasty on the function of the Eustachian tube in children with cleft palate. Cleft Palate J. 1986;23:63–8.
13. Boston M, McCook J, Burke B, Derkay C. Incidence of and risk factors for additional tympanostomy tube insertion in children. Arch Otolaryngol Head Neck Surg. 2003;129:293–6.
14. Poelmans J, Tack J, Feesnstra L. Chronic middle ear disease and gastroesophageal reflux disease: a causal relation? Otol Neurotol. 2001;22:447–50.
15. White DR, Heavner SB, Hardy SM, Prazma J. Gastroesophageal reflux and Eustachian tube dysfunction in animal model. Laryngoscope. 2002;112:955–61.
16. Rozmanic V, Volepic M, Athel V, Bonifacic D, Velepic M. Prolonged esophageal pH monitoring in the evaluation of gastroesophageal reflux in children with chronic tubotympanal disorders. J Pediatr Gastroenterol Nutr. 2002;34:278–80.
17. Tasker A, Dettmar PW, Panetti M, Koufman JA, Birchall JP, Pearson JP. Reflux of gastric juice and glue ear in children. Lancet. 2002;359:493.
18. Tasker A, Dettmar PW, Panetti M, Koufman JA, Birchall JP, Pearson JP. Is gastric reflux a cause of otitis media with effusion in children? Laryngoscope. 2002;112:1930–4.
19. Antonelli PJ, Lloyd KM, Lee JC. Gastric reflux is uncommon in acute post-tympanostomy otorrhea. Otolaryngol Head Neck Surg. 2005;132:523–6.
20. Pitkaranta A, Kalho KL, Rautelin H. Helicobacter pylori in children who are prone to upper respiratory tract infections. Arch Otolaryng Head Neck Surg. 2005;131:256–8.
21. Miura MS, Mascaro M, Rosenfeld RM. Association between otitis media and gastroesophageal reflux: a systematic review. Otolaryngol Head Neck Surg. 2012;146:354–52.
22. Howie VM, Plousard JH. Bacterial etiology and antimicrobial treatment of exudative otitis media: relation of antibiotic therapy to relapses. South Med J. 1971;64:233–9.
23. Pillsbury HC 3rd, Kveton JF, Sasaki CT, Frazier W. Quantitative bacteriology in adenoid tissue. Otolaryngol Head Neck Surg. 1981;89:355–63.
24. Gates GA, Avery CA, Prihoda TJ, Cooper JC Jr. Effectiveness of adenoidectomy and tympanostomy tubes in the treatment of chronic otitis media with effusion. N Engl J Med. 1987;317:1444–51.
25. Maw R, Bawden R. Spontaneous resolution of severe chronic glue ear in children and the effect of adenoidectomy, tonsillectomy and insertion of ventilation tubes (grommets). BMJ. 1993;306:756–60.
26. Paradise JL, Bluestone CD, Rogers KD, Taylor FH, Colborn DK, Bochman RZ, et al. Efficacy of adenoidectomy for recurrent otitis media in children previously treated with tympanostomy tube placement. Results of parallel randomized and nonrandomized trials. JAMA. 1990;263:2066–73.
27. Paradise JL, Bluestone CD, Colborn DK, Bernard BS, Smith CG, Rockette HE, et al. Adenoidectomy and adenotonsillectomy for recurrent acute otitis media: parallel randomized clinical trial in children not previously treated with tympanostomy tubes. JAMA. 1999;282:945–53.
28. Kouvunem P, Uhari M, Luotonen J, Kristo A, Rask R, Pokka T, et al. Adenoidectomy versus chemoprophylaxis and placebo for recurrent acute otitis media in children aged under 2 years: randomised controlled trial. BMJ. 2004;328:487–91.
29. Mattilla OS, Joki-Erkkila VP, Kilpi T, Jokinen J, Herva E, Phakka H. Prevention of otitis media by adenoidectomy in children younger than 2 years. Arch Otolaryngol Head Neck Surg. 2003;129:163–8.
30. Gates GA, Avery CA, Cooper JC Jr, Prihoda TJ. Chronic secretory otitis media: effects of surgical management. Ann Otol Rhinol Laryngol. 1989;138:2–32.
31. Homoe P, Christensen RB, Bretlau P. Acute otitis media and sociomedical risk factors among unselected children in Greenland. Int J Pediatric Otorhinolaryngol. 1999;49:37–52.
32. Lim DJ, Hermansson A, Ryan AF, et al. Panel 4: recent advances in otitis media in molecular biology, biochemistry, genetics, and animal models. Otolaryngol Head Neck Surg. 2013;114(Suppl 4):E52–63.
33. Kalm O, Johnson U, Prellner K, Ninn K. HLA. frequency in patients with recurrent acute otitis media. Arch Otolaryngol Head Neck Surg. 1991;117:1296–9.
34. Kvaerner KJ, Tambs K, Harris JR, Magnus P. Distribution and heritability of recurrent ear infections. Ann Otol Rhinol Laryngol. 1997;106:624–32.

35. Rovers M, Haggard M, Gannon M, et al. Heritability of symptom domains in otitis media: a longitudinal study of 1373 twin pairs. Am J Epidemiol. 2002;155:958–64.
36. Casselbrant ML, Mandel EM, Fall PA, et al. The heritability of otitis media: a twin and triplet study. JAMA. 1999;282:2125–30.
37. Casselbrant ML, Mandel EM, Rockette HE, et al. The genetic component of middle ear disease in the first 5 years of life. Arch Otolaryngol Head Neck Surg. 2004;130:273–8.
38. Daly KA, Brown WM, Segade F, Bowden DW, Keats B, Lindgren BR, Levine SC, Rich SS. Chronic and recurrent otitis media: a genome scan for susceptibility loci. Am J Hum Genet. 2004;75:988–97.
39. Casselbrant ML, Mandel EM, Jung J, Ferrel RE, Tekely K, Szatkiewicz JP, Ray A, Weeks DE. Otitis media: a genome-wide linkage scan with evidence of susceptibility loci within the 17q12 and 10q22.3 regions. BMC Med Genet. 2009;10:85–94.
40. Castagno LA, Lavinsky L. Otitis media in children: seasonal changes and socioeconomic level. Int J Pediatr Otorhinolaryngol. 2002;62:129–34.
41. Casselbrant ML, Brostoff LM, Cantekin EI, Flaherty MR, Doyle WJ, Bluestone CD, et al. Otitis media with effusion in preschool children. Laryngoscope. 1985;95:428–36.
42. Van Cauwenberge PB. Relevant and irrelevant predisposing factors in secretory otitis media. Acta Otolaryngol Suppl. 1984;414:147–53.
43. Alho OP, Oja H, Koivu M, Sorri M. Risk factor for chronic otitis media with effusion in infancy. Each acute otitis media episode induces a high but transient risk. Arch Otolaryngol Head Neck Surg. 1995;121:839–43.
44. Revai K, Dobbs LA, Nair S, Patel JA, Grady JJ, Chonmaitree T. Incidence of acute otitis media and sinusitis complicating upper respiratory tract infection: the effect of age. Pediatrics. 2007;119:1408–12.
45. Chonmaitreee T, Revai K, Grady JJ, Clos A, Janak AP, Nair S, Fan J, Henrickson KJ. Viral upper respiratory tract infection and otitis media complication in young children. Clin Infect Dis. 2008;46:815–23.
46. Winther B, Alper CM, Mandel EM, Doyle WJ, Hendley JO. Temporal relationships between colds, upper respiratory viruses detected by polymerase chain reaction, and otitis media in young children followed through a typical cold season. Pediatrics 2007;119:1069–75.
47. Sarkkinen H, Ruuskanen O, Meuman O, Phakkat H, Virolainen E, Eskola J. Identification of respiratory virus antigen in middle ear fluids of children with acute otitis media. J Infec Dis. 1985;151:444–8.
48. Klein BS, Dolletttem FR, Youlkenm RH. The role of respiratory syncytial virus and other viral pathogens in acute otitis media. J Pediatr. 1982;101:16–20.
49. Buchman CA, Doyle WJ, Skoner D, Fireman P, Gwaltney JM. Otologic manifestations of experimental rhinovirus infection. Laryngoscope. 1994;104:1295–9.
50. Bylander A. Upper respiratory tract infection and Eustachian tube dysfunction in children. Acta Otolaryngol. 1984;97:343–9.
51. Alho OP, Koivu M, Sorri M, Rantakallio P. Risk factor for recurrent acute otitis media and respiratory infection in infancy. Int J Pediatr Otorhinolaryngol. 1990;19:151–61.
52. Fiellau-Nikolajasen M. Tympanometry in three-year-old children. Type of care as an epidemiologic factor in secretory otitis media and tubal dysfunction in unselected populations of three-year old children. ORL J Otorhinolaryngol Relat Spec. 1979;41:193–205.
53. Tos M, Poulsen G, Borch J. Tympanometry in 2-year-old children. ORL J Otorhinolaryngol Relat Spec. 1978;40:77–85.
54. Côté SM, Peticlerc A, Rynault MF, et al. Short- and long-term risk of infections as a function of group child care attendance: a 8-year population-based study. Arch Pediatr Adolesc Med. 2010;164:1132–7.
55. Wald ER, Dashefsky B, Byers C, Guerra N, Taylor F. Frequency and severity of infections in day care. J Pediatr. 1988;112:540–6.
56. Alho OP, Läärä E, Oja H. Public health impact of various risk factors for acute otitis media in northern Finland. Am J Epidemiol. 1996;143:1149–56.
57. Ladomenou F, Kafatos A, Tselentis Y, Galanakis E. Predisposing factor for acute otitis media in infancy. J Infect. 2010;61:49–53.
58. Lim DJ. Recent advances in otitis media with effusion. Report of the Fourth Research Conference. Ann Otol Rhinol Laryngol. 1989;98(Suppl 139):10–55.
59. Daly KA, Rich SS, Levine S, Margolis RH, Le CT, Lidgren B, et al. The family study of otitis media: design and disease and risk factor profiles. Genet Epidemiol. 1996;13:451–68.
60. Daly KA, Brown JE, Lindgren BR, Meland MH, Le CT, Giebink GS. Epidemiology of otitis media onset by six months of age. Pediatrics. 1999;103:1158–66.
61. Vinther B, Elbrond O, Pedersen B. A population study of otitis media in childhood. Acta Otolaryngol Suppl. 1979;360:135–7.
62. Teele DW, Klein JO, Rosner B, Greater Boston Otitis Media Study Group. Epidemiology of otitis media during the first seven years of life in children in greater Boston: a prospective cohort study. J Infect Dis. 1989;160:83–94.
63. Stratchan DP, Cook DG. Health effects of passive smoking. 4. Parental smoking, middle ear disease and adenotonsillectomy in children. Thorax. 1998;53:50–6.
64. Strenstrom R, Bernard PA, Bem-Simhon H. Exposure to environmental tobacco smoke as a risk factor for recurrent acute otitis media in children under the age of five years. Int J Pediatr Otorhinolaryngol. 1993;27:127–36.
65. Kitchens GG. Relationship of environmental tobacco smoke to otitis media in young children. Laryngoscope. 1995;105:1–13.
66. Blakley BW, Blakley JE. Smoking and middle ear disease: are they related? A review article. Otolaryngol Head Neck Surg. 1995;112:441–6.

67. Birch L, Elbrond O. A prospective epidemiological study of secretory otitis media in young children related to the indoor environment. ORL J Otorhinolaryngol Relat Spec. 1987;49:253–8.

68. Hinton AE, Buckley G. Parental smoking and middle ear effusion in children. J Laryngol Otol. 1988;102:992–6.

69. Lubianca Neto JF, Burns AG, Lu L, Mombach R, Saffer M. Passive smoking and non-recurrent acute otitis media in children. Otolaryngol Head Neck Surg. 1999;121:805–8.

70. Zielhuis GA, Rach GH, Van Den Broekm P. Predisposing factors for otitis media with effusion in young children. Adv Otorhinolaryngol. 1988;40:65–9.

71. Owen MJ, Baldwin CD, Swank PR, Pannu AK, Johnson DL, Howie VM. Relation of infant feeding practices, cigarette smoke exposure, and group child care to the onset and duration of otitis media with effusion in the first two years of life. J Pediatr.1993;123:702–11.

72. Ey JL, Holberg CJ, Aldous MB, Wright A, Martinez FD, Taussig LM. Passive smoke exposure and otitis media in the first year of life. Pediatrics. 1995;95:670–7.

73. Collet JP, Larson CP, Boivin JF, Suissa S, Pless IB. Parental smoking and risk of otitis media in pre-school children. Can J POublic Health. 1995;86:269–73.

74. Hammaren-Malmi S, Saxen H, Tarkkanen J, Mattila PS. Passive smoking after tympanostomy and risk of recurrent acute otitis media. Int J Pediatr Otorhinolaryngol. 2007;71:1305–10.

75. Etzel RA. Smoke and ear effusions. Pediatrics. 1987;79:309–11.

76. Ilicali OC, Keles N, Deer K, Asum OF, Guidiken Y. Evaluation of the effect of passive smoking on otitis media in children by an objective method: urinary cotinine analysis. Laryngoscope. 2001;11:163–7.

77. Uhari M, Mottonen M. An open randomized controlled trial of infection prevention in child day-care centers. Pediatr Infect Dis J. 1999;18:672–7.

78. Saarinen UM. Prolonged breast feeding as prophylaxis for recurrent otitis media. Acta Pediatr Scand. 1982;71:567–71.

79. Cunningham AS. Morbidity in breast-fed and artificially fed infants. II. J Pediatr. 1979;95:685–9.

80. Chandra RK. Prospective studies of the effect of breast feeding on incidence of infection and allergy. Acta Pediatr Scand. 1982;71:567–71.

81. Duncan RB. Positional otitis media. Arch Otolaryngol. 1960;72:454–63.

82. Duffy LC, Faden H, Wasielewski R, Wolf J, Krystofik D. Exclusive breastfeeding protects against bacterial colonization and day care exposure to otitis media. Pediatrics. 1997;100:E7.

83. Mandel EM, Doyle WJ, Winther B, Alper CM. The incidence, prevalence and burden of OM in unselected children aged 1-8years followed by weekly otoscopy through the "common cold" season. Int J Pediatr Otorhinolaryngol. 2008;72:491–9.

84. Harsten G, Prellner K, Heldrup J, Kalm O, Kornfalt R. Recurrent acute otitis media. A prospective study of children during the first three years of life. Acta Otolaryngol. 1989;107:11–9.

85. Tainio V, Savilahti E, Salmenpera L, Arjomaa P, Siimes MA, Perheentupa J. Risk factors for infantile recurrent otitis media: atopy but not type of feeding. Pediatr Res. 1988;23:509–12.

86. Beauregard RB. Positional otitis media. J Pediatr. 1971;79:294–6.

87. Sassen ML, Brand R, Grote JJ. Breast-feeding and acute otitis media. Am J Otolaryngol. 1994;15:351–7.

88. Niemela M, Uhari M, Hannuksela A. Pacifiers and dental structure as risk factors for otitis media. Int J Pediatr Otorhinolaryngol. 1994;29:121–7.

89. Niemela M, Uhari M, Mötönen M. A pacifier increases the risk of recurrent acute otitis media in children in day-care centers. Pediatrics. 1995;96:884–8.

90. Niemela M, Phakari O, Pokka T, Uhari M. Pacifier as a risk factor for acute otitis media: a randomized controlled trial of parental counseling. Pediatrics. 2000;106:483–8.

91. Warren JJ, Levy SM, Kirchner HL, Nowak AJ, Bergus GR. Pacifier use and the occurrence of otitis media in the first year of life. Pediatr Dent. 2001;23:103–7.

Microbiology, Antimicrobial Susceptibility, and Antibiotic Treatment

5

Tania Sih and Rita Krumenaur

Introduction

Otitis media (OM) is caused by respiratory virus and/or bacterial infection of the middle ear space and the resulting host response to infection [1]. Acute otitis media (AOM) occurs most frequently as a consequence of viral upper respiratory tract infection (URTI) [2–4], which leads to eustachian tube inflammation/dysfunction, negative middle ear pressure, and movement of secretions containing the URTI-causative virus and pathogenic bacteria in the nasopharynx into the middle ear cleft. By using comprehensive and sensitive microbiologic testing, bacteria and/or viruses can be detected in the middle ear fluid (MEF) in up to 96 % of AOM cases (e.g., 66 % bacteria and viruses together, 27 % bacteria alone, and 4 % virus alone) [5]. Studies using less sensitive or less comprehensive microbiologic assays have yielded less positive results for bacteria and much less positive results for viruses [6–8].

Microbiology

Virus

Epidemiologic studies have shown a strong relationship between viral upper respiratory infections (URIs) and AOM. Chonmaitree et al. reported that 63 % of 864 URI episodes of children less than 4 years of age in the USA were positive for respiratory viruses and adenovirus, coronavirus, and respiratory syncytial virus (RSV) frequently related to AOM [4].

In children with AOM in Japan, respiratory viruses were detected in 35 % of patients ($n = 1092$). RSV, influenza virus, and adenovirus were of the most common viruses [9]. Grieves et al. [10, 11] studied RSV pathogenesis in chinchillas to investigate how viral URI leads to AOM. After nasal RSV challenge, viral replication was seen from the site of inoculation to the pharyngeal orifice of the eustachian tube by 48 h, and the virus could be detected in the distal part of the eustachian tube after 5 days.

RSV and adenoviruses are still among the most important viruses associated with AOM. In a prospective, longitudinal study of children younger than 4 years in the USA, 63 % of 864 URI episodes were positive for respiratory viruses; rhinovirus and adenovirus were most frequently detected [4]. Of URI caused by a single virus, the rate of AOM complicating URI was highest in the episodes caused by adenovirus, coronavirus, and RSV.

T. Sih (✉)
Department of Pediatric Otolaryngology, Medical School University of São Paulo, São Paulo 01239-040, Brazil
e-mail: tsih@amcham.com.br

R. Krumenaur
Department of Pediatric Otolaryngology,
Santo Antonio Hospital for Children, Porto Alegre, Brazil

© Springer International Publishing Switzerland 2015
D. Preciado (ed.), *Otitis Media: State of the art concepts and treatment*, DOI 10.1007/978-3-319-17888-2_5

Molecular technologies have made it possible to detect new respiratory viruses related with AOM. Human metapneumoviruses (hMPV) were discovered a decade ago, and are now recognized as an important pathogen causing lower respiratory tract infection and URTIs in children. In a cohort of 1338 children with respiratory symptoms, hMPV was detected in 3.5% of the children, and 41% of infections were complicated by AOM [12]. The incidence of hMPV was highest in children younger than 2 years (7.6%); 61% of children younger than 3 years of age had hMPV infections complicated by AOM.

Human bocavirus (hBoV) was discovered in 2005; to date, the significance of hBoV in causing symptomatic illness is still controversial. hBoV occurs frequently in conjunction with other viruses and seems to persist for a long time in the respiratory tract. In asymptomatic children, hBoV has been detected from respiratory specimens at an alarmingly high rate (43–44%) [13, 14]. In children with AOM, Beder et al. [15] have reported an hBoV detection rate of 6.3% from nasopharyngeal secretions (NPS) and 2.7% from MEF. The resolution time of AOM was longer, and the rate of fever was higher in children with hBoV. The virus has also been detected from 3% of the MEFs from young children with otitis media with effusion (OME) [16]. The role of this virus in AOM and OME requires further investigation.

The new and old picornaviruses have also been studied in association with AOM. In young children with AOM, a new rhinovirus, human rhinovirus species C (HRV-C), was detected in almost half of the rhinovirus-positive NPS and MEF samples [17].

In a study of 495 children with AOM in Japan, Yano et al. [18] found 12 (2.4%) cases with cytomegalovirus (CMV) infection; five of these cases (3–25 months of age) were primary CMV infection or reactivation documented by immunoglobulin M (IgM) serology [18]. Four of these five had CMV or viral nucleic acids in the MEF; two of five had no bacteria cultured from the MEF. The investigators suggested the role of CMV in AOM etiology. Similar findings have previously been reported. Because CMV is a rare cause of viral URI in young children, it is likely that the contribution of this virus to AOM is limited although possible.

Viral–Bacterial Interactions

Pathogenesis of AOM involves complex interactions between viruses and bacteria; acute viral infection of the nasopharynx creates the environment that promotes the growth of pathogenic bacteria, which already colonize the nasopharynx and promote their adhesion to the epithelial cells and invasion into the middle ear.

Symptoms of viral URTIs usually last for a week, and viral shedding from the nasopharynx may last 3 weeks or longer. Studies of viral persistence in the nasopharynx, viral transmission, and asymptomatic infections have become more important in understanding the pathogenesis of URI and AOM. Viral infections from the upper respiratory tract usually induce major or minor damages of respiratory mucosa following the promotion of the growth of pathogenic bacteria in the nasopharynx, the enhancement of bacterial adhesion to the epithelial cells, and the eventual invasion into the middle ear causing AOM.

Ishizuka et al. reported that rhinovirus infecting cultured human airway epithelial cells stimulated *Streptococcus pneumoniae* adhesion to airway epithelial cells via increases in platelet-activating receptor (PAF-R) [19]. Increased adherence of *S. pneumoniae* may be one of the reasons that AOM or pneumonia develops after rhinovirus infections by inducing surface expression of PAF-R, a receptor for *S. pneumoniae* [20, 21]. In a mouse model, Sendai virus coinfection with *S. pneumoniae* and *Moraxella catarrhalis* increased the incidence rate, duration of AOM, and bacterial load [22].

In the human study, the detection of rhinovirus or adenovirus in the nasopharynx was positively associated with the presence of *Haemophilus influenzae* (aboriginal children) and *M. catarrhalis* (aboriginal and nonaboriginal children). However, adenovirus was negatively associated with *S. pneumoniae* in aboriginal children [23]. Tomochika et al. reported from Japan that 31 % of hospitalized children with RSV had AOM [24].

RSV nasal inoculation in chinchillas reduced the expression of the antimicrobial peptide chinchilla b-defensin 1 and increased the load of *H. influenzae* in the nasopharynx [25]. Infection of the airway with a respiratory virus downregulates the expression of b-defensin, which increases the nasopharyngeal colonization with *H. influenzae* and further promotes the development of AOM.

Bacteriology

The gold standard in determining the etiology of bacterial OM is the culture of MEF. In order to determine the OM bacteriology, the culture of MEF is recovered by tympanocentesis, drainage from tympanostomy tubes, or spontaneous otorrhea. These determinations are important to track changes in the distribution of pathogens that cause OM.

Bacteria are found in 50–90 % of cases of AOM with or without otorrhea [26]. *S. pneumoniae*, nontypeable *H. influenzae* or *M. catarrhalis* are the leading causative pathogens responsible for AOM, and they frequently colonize in the nasopharynx [26]. *Streptococcus pyogenes* (group A β-hemolytic streptococci) accounts for less than 5 % of AOM cases. The proportion of AOM cases with pathogenic bacteria isolated from the MEF varies depending on bacteriologic techniques, transport issues, and stringency of AOM definition. In series of reports from the USA and Europe from 1952–1981 and 1985–1992, the mean percentage of cases with bacterial pathogens isolated from the MEFs was 69 and 72 %, respectively [26]. A large series from the University of Pittsburgh Otitis Media Study Group reported bacterial pathogens in 84 % of the MEFs from 2807 cases of AOM [26]. Studies that applied more stringent otoscopic criteria and/or use of bedside specimen plating on solid agar in addition to liquid transport media have a reported rate of recovery of pathogenic bacteria from middle ear exudates ranging from 85 to 90 % [27–29]. When using appropriate stringent diagnostic criteria, careful specimen handling, and sensitive microbiologic techniques, the vast majority of cases of AOM involve pathogenic bacteria either alone or in concert with viral pathogens.

Clinical bacteriology has dramatically changed after the introduction of pneumococcal conjugate vaccine (PCV) [30]. The most commonly identified pathogen is *S. pneumonia*, which, prior to adoption of the 7-valent pneumococcal conjugate vaccine (PCV7), was isolated in approximately one third to half of all cases [30]. Block et al. studied changes of microbiology after the community-wide vaccination with PCV7 [31]. Comparing each cohort (1992–1998 vs. 2000–2003), the proportion of *S. pneumoniae* significantly decreased from 48 to 31 %, and nontypable *H. influenzae* significantly increased from 41 to 56 %. Post-PCV7, Gram-negative bacteria and beta-lactamase-producing organisms accounted for two thirds and one half of all AOM isolates, respectively. In terms of serotypic change in *S. pneumoniae*, vaccine efficacy of PCV7 against vaccine-serotype pneumococcal OM was about 60 %. A later report [32] with data from 2007 to 2009, 6–8 years after the introduction of PCV7 in the USA, showed that PCV7 strains of *S. pneumoniae* virtually disappeared from the MEF of children with AOM who had been vaccinated. However, the frequency of isolation of non-PCV7 serotypes of *S. pneumoniae* from the MEF overall increased; this has made isolation of *S. pneumoniae* and *H. influenzae* of children with AOM nearly equal. In summary, the licensed 7-valent CRM197-PCV7 has modest beneficial effects in healthy infants with a low baseline risk of AOM. Administering PCV7 in high-risk infants, after early infancy and in older children with a history of AOM, appears to have no benefit in preventing further episodes.

Serotype 19A was a major cause of replacement disease following introduction of PCV7 [32–34]. Over the past decade, serotype 19A emerged as a major cause of acute OM, recurrent OM, and severe mastoiditis [32–34]. The increase in 19A was often attributed to introduction of PCV7. However, Dagan et al. [35] described the emergence of serotype 19A as a cause of OM prior to the introduction of PCV7 in Israel. Analysis of antibiotic administration patterns suggests that antibiotic use may contribute to the emergence of certain lineages of *S. pneumoniae* [36, 37].

In 2010, a pneumococcal vaccine with 13 serotypes (1, 3, 4, 5, 6A, 6B, 7F, 9V, 14, 18C, 19A, 19F and 23F) conjugated to diphtheria protein was licensed. PC-13V utilizes the same protein carrier as vaccine PC-7V, and was released in the United States by the FDA on the basis of immunogenicity and safety studies. Safety was evaluated by means of 13 controlled studies involving thousands of healthy children. It is still early to evaluate the true benefit of PVC 13, and numerous trials are under development. PC-13V is recommended for all children between 2 and 59 months of age and those between 5 and 6 years with risk factors for severe pneumococcal disease. The vaccine is applied in 4 doses at 2, 4, 6 and 12 months of age.

Currently, several RCTs with different (newly licensed, multivalent) PCVs administered during early infancy are ongoing to establish their effects on AOM. Results of these studies may provide a better understanding of the role of the newly licensed, multivalent PCVs in preventing AOM.

In a study of tympanocentesis over four respiratory tract illness seasons in a private practice, the percentage of *S. pneumoniae* initially decreased relative to *H. influenzae*. In 2005–2006 ($N=33$), 48% of bacteria were *S. pneumoniae*, and 42% were *H. influenzae*. For 2006–2007 ($N=37$), the percentages were equal at 41%. In 2007–2008 ($N=34$), 35% were *S. pneumoniae*, and 59% were *H. influenzae*. In 2008–2009 ($N=24$), the percentages were 54% and 38%, respectively, with an increase in intermediate and nonsusceptible *S. pneumoniae* [38]. Data on nasopharyngeal colonization from PCV7-immunized children with AOM have shown continued presence of *S. pneumoniae* colonization. Revai et al. [39] showed no difference in *S. pneumoniae* colonization rate among children with AOM who have been unimmunized, under-immunized, or fully immunized with PCV7. In a study during a viral URTI, including mostly PCV7-immunized children (6 months to 3 years of age), *S. pneumoniae* was detected in 45.5%

of 968 nasopharyngeal swabs, *H. influenzae* was detected in 32.4%, and *M. catarrhalis* was detected in 63.1% [40]. Data show that nasopharyngeal colonization of children vaccinated with PCV7 increasingly is caused by *S. pneumoniae* serotypes not contained in the vaccine [41–44]. With the use of the recently licensed 13-valent pneumococcal conjugate vaccine (PCV13) [45], the patterns of nasopharyngeal colonization and infection with these common AOM bacterial pathogens will continue to evolve.

Investigators have attempted to predict the type of AOM pathogenic bacteria on the basis of clinical severity, but the results have not been promising. *S. pyogenes* has been shown to occur more commonly in older children [46] and cause a greater degree of inflammation of the middle ear and tympanic membrane (TM), a greater frequency of spontaneous rupture of the TM, and more frequent progression to acute mastoiditis compared with other bacterial pathogens [46–48]. As for clinical findings in cases with *S. pneumoniae* and nontypeable *H. influenzae*, some studies suggest that signs and symptoms of AOM caused by *S. pneumoniae* may be more severe (fever, severe earache, bulging TM) than those caused by other pathogens [29, 49, 50]. These findings were refuted by results of the studies that found AOM caused by nontypeable *H. influenzae* to be associated with bilateral AOM and more severe inflammation of the TM [51, 52]. Leibovitz et al. [53] concluded, in a study of 372 children with AOM caused by *H. influenzae* ($N=138$), *S. pneumoniae* ($N=64$), and mixed *H. influenzae* and *S. pneumoniae* ($N=64$), that clinical/otologic scores could not discriminate among various bacterial etiologies of AOM. However, there were significantly different clinical/otologic scores between bacterial culture-negative and culture-positive cases. A study of middle ear exudates of 82 cases of bullous myringitis has shown a 97% bacteria-positive rate, primarily *S. pneumoniae*. In contrast to the previous belief, *Mycoplasma* sp. is rarely the causative agent in this condition [54]. Accurate prediction of the bacterial cause of AOM on the basis of clinical presentation, without bacterial culture of the middle ear exudates, is not possible, but specific etiologies may be predicted in some situations. Published evidence has suggested that AOM associated with conjunctivitis (otitis-conjunctivitis syndrome) is more likely caused by nontypeable *H. influenzae* than by other bacteria [55–57].

M. catarrhalis is derived from the upper respiratory tract [58]. High rate of spontaneous clinical resolution occurs in children with AOM attributable to *M. catarrhalis* [59, 60]. AOM attributable to *M. catarrhalis* rarely progresses to acute mastoiditis or intracranial infections [61, 62].

Substantial geographic variability is observed in the proportion of OM caused by *M. catarrhalis*. For example, the rate of *M.catarrhalis* in Israel is low, whereas in Finland this microorganism is the most common bacterial cause of recurrent OM in children with tympanostomy tubes [63, 64]. As the distribution of pathogens changes with widespread use of PCVs, the relative proportion of OM due to *M. catarrhalis* is increasing in some studies [65, 66].

Polymicrobial Interactions

A murine model of nasal colonization and AOM to study relationships among various combinations of bacterial OM pathogens (*S. pneumoniae*, *H. influenzae*, and *M. catarrhalis*) and Sendai virus, which is the murine equivalent of human parainfluenza virus has been reported by Krishnamurthy et al. [22]. As expected, viral infection significantly increased the incidence of acute OM. Coinfections with *S. pneumoniae* and *M. catarrhalis* increased the incidence and duration of pneumococcal OM compared with *S. pneumoniae* alone and *S. pneumoniae* and *H. influenzae* together.

Host competition may also affect the selection of virulence characteristics in *S. pneumoniae* [67]. A combination of theoretical models and in vivo nasopharyngeal colonization experiments was used to demonstrate that competition with *H. influenzae* may select for more virulent strains of *S. pneumoniae*.

Taken as a whole, the studies indicated that the specific combination of colonizing bacteria

and respiratory viruses can alter the incidence and duration of OM, and pneumococci have several methods to compete with co-colonizing and coinfecting species.

Implications of Bacterial Vaccine Efforts for Practice

The recurrent nature of acute otitis media continues to be burdensome to children and families, especially those who suffer from frequent recurrences and in disadvantaged populations where disease progresses to chronic suppurative otitis media with associated impacts on hearing loss and educational potential. PC-7V has reduced the burden of vaccine-serotype disease as well as shifted the pneumococcal serotypes carried in the nasopharynx toward those with lower disease-causing potential. Antibiotic resistance remains a challenge to successful therapy with ceftriaxone-resistant pneumococci present in the community and increasing emergence of b-lactamase–negative, amoxicillin-resistant NTHi identified globally. The next-generation PC-13V has been introduced, and early data suggest efficacy against invasive pneumococcal disease and carriage of SP19A, the multidrug resistance isolate that has been associated with both treatment failure in AOM 90 and the increasing number of cases of pneumococcal mastoiditis. Promising data on an 11-valent pneumococcal polysaccharide conjugate vaccine with protein D as a carrier was published in 2006, but additional confirmation of efficacy against NTHi otitis media with the licensed formulation, PHiD-CV (a 10-valent conjugate), is pending data future studies. For NTHI specifically, a number of candidate protein antigens have had progress to human trials since 2007, remains to be demonstrated. Multiple candidates have demonstrated the necessary requirements for candidate vaccine antigens: conservation among isolates, surface exposure, immunogenicity in animals, and protection in animal models of disease or specifically experimental otitis media. Further research of the role of each antigen in the pathogenesis of disease, to elicit response in the youngest infants is likely to be productive and permit more antigens to move into clinical trials.

Bacterial Susceptibility to Antibiotics

Selection of antibiotic to treat AOM is based on the suspected type of bacteria and antibiotic susceptibility pattern, although clinical pharmacology and clinical and microbiologic results and predicted compliance with the drug are also taken into account. Early studies of AOM patients show that 19% of children with *S. pneumoniae* and 48% with *H. influenzae* cultured on initial tympanocentesis who were not treated with antibiotic cleared the bacteria at the time of a second tympanocentesis 2–7 days later [68]. Approximately 75% of children infected with *M. catarrhalis* experienced bacteriologic cure even after treatment with amoxicillin, an antibiotic to which it is not susceptible [59, 60].

Antibiotic susceptibility of major AOM bacterial pathogens continues to change, but data on middle ear pathogens have become scanty because tympanocentesis is not generally performed in studies of children with uncomplicated AOM. Most available data come from cases of persistent or recurrent AOM. Current US data from a number of centers indicate that approximately 83 and 87% of isolates of *S. pneumoniae* from all age groups are susceptible to regular (40 mg/kg/day) and high-dose (80–90 mg/kg/day divided twice daily) amoxicillin, respectively [69–73]. Pediatric isolates are smaller in number and include mostly ear isolates collected from recurrent and persistent AOM cases with a high percentage of multidrug-resistant *S. pneumoniae*, most frequently nonvaccine serotypes that have recently increased in frequency and importance [37].

The definitions of resistance are the minimum inhibitory concentration (MIC) breakpoints set by the Clinical and Laboratory Standards Institute (CLSI). CLSI has established a new approach to penicillin breakpoints [74], and this approach is needed to guide appropriate treatment because it takes into account whether penicillin is given orally or parenterally, and whether the patient has meningitis. The revised penicillin breakpoints are for infections other than meningitis. Currently, the studies of AOM use the new oral penicillin breakpoints and define all isolates with a penicillin MIC of ≤ 2.0 μg/mL as penicillin nonsusceptible *S. pneumoniae* (PNSP), or use an MIC of 4.0 μg/mL to define penicillin-intermediately resistant *S. pneumoniae* (PISP), and ≥ 8.0 μg/mL to define penicillin-resistant *S. pneumoniae* (PRSP).

High-dose amoxicillin will yield MEF levels that exceed the MIC of all *S. pneumoniae* serotypes that are intermediately (penicillin MIC 4.0 μg/mL) and, many but not all, highly resistant serotypes (penicillin MIC ≥ 8.0 μg/mL) for a longer period of the dosing interval and has been shown to improve bacteriologic and clinical efficacy compared with the regular dose [75, 76]. Hoberman et al. [77] reported superior efficacy of high-dose amoxicillin/clavulanate in eradication of *S. pneumoniae* (96%) from the middle ear at days 4 to 6 of therapy compared with azithromycin.

The antibiotic susceptibility pattern for *S. pneumoniae* is expected to continue to evolve with the use of PCV13, a conjugate vaccine containing 13 serotypes of *S. pneumoniae* [78–80]. Widespread use of PCV13 could potentially reduce diseases caused by multidrug-resistant pneumococcal serotypes and diminish the need for the use of higher dose of amoxicillin or amoxicillin/clavulanate for AOM. Some *H. influenzae* isolates produce β-lactamase enzyme, causing the isolate to become resistant to penicillins. Current data from different studies with non-AOM sources and geographic locations that may not be comparable show that 58–82% of *H. influenzae* isolates are susceptible to regular and high-dose amoxicillin [42, 70, 71, 81]. These data represented a significant decrease in β-lactamase-producing *H. influenzae*, compared with data reported in the 2004 AOM guideline.

Nationwide data suggest that 100% of *M. catarrhalis* derived from the upper respiratory tract are β-lactamase-positive but remain susceptible to amoxicillin-clavulanate [81]. However, the high rate of spontaneous clinical resolution occurring in children with AOM attributable to *M.*

catarrhalis treated with amoxicillin reduces the concern for the first-line coverage for this microorganism [59, 60]. AOM attributable to *M. catarrhalis* rarely progresses to acute mastoiditis or intracranial infections [62, 82, 83].

Antibiotic Therapy

High-dose amoxicillin is recommended as the first-line treatment in most patients, although there are a number of medications that are clinically effective [1]. The justification for the use of amoxicillin relates to its effectiveness against common AOM bacterial pathogens as well as its safety, low cost, acceptable taste, and narrow microbiologic spectrum [59, 75]. In children who have taken amoxicillin in the previous 30 days, those with concurrent conjunctivitis, or those or whom coverage for β-lactamase-positive *H. influenzae* and *M. catarrhalis* is desired, therapy should be initiated with high-dose amoxicillin/clavulanate (90 mg/kg/day of amoxicillin, with 6.4 mg/kg/day of clavulanate, a ratio of amoxicillin to clavulanate of 14:1, given in two divided doses, which is less likely to cause diarrhea than other amoxicillin/clavulanate preparations) [84].

Alternative initial antibiotics include cefdinir (14 mg/kg per day in one or two doses), cefuroxime (30 mg/kg per day in two divided doses), cefpodoxime (10 mg/kg per day in two divided doses), or ceftriaxone (50 mg/kg, administered intramuscularly). It is important to note that alternative antibiotics vary in their efficacy against AOM pathogens. For example, recent US data on in vitro susceptibility of *S. pneumoniae* to cefdinir and cefuroxime are 70–80%, compared with 84–92% amoxicillin efficacy [69–72]. In vitro efficacy of cefdinir and cefuroxime against *H. influenzae* is approximately 98%, compared with 58% efficacy of amoxicillin and nearly 100% efficacy of amoxicillin/clavulanate [81]. A multicenter double tympanocentesis open-label study of cefdinir in recurrent AOM attributable to *H. influenzae* showed eradication of the organism in 72% of patients [85].

For penicillin-allergic children, recent data suggest that cross-reactivity among penicillins and cephalosporins is lower than historically reported [86–89]. The previously cited rate of cross-sensitivity to cephalosporins among penicillin-allergic patients (approximately 10%) is likely an overestimate. The rate was based on data collected and reviewed during the 1960s and 1970s. A study analyzing pooled data of 23 studies, including 2400 patients with reported history of penicillin allergy and 39,000 with no penicillin-allergic history concluded that many patients who present with a history of penicillin allergy do not have an immunologic reaction to penicillin [88]. The chemical structure of the cephalosporin determines the risk of cross-reactivity between specific agents [87, 90]. The degree of cross-reactivity is higher between penicillins and first-generation cephalosporins but is negligible with the second-and third-generation cephalosporins. Because of the differences in the chemical structures, cefdinir, cefuroxime, cefpodoxime, and ceftriaxone are highly unlikely to be associated with cross-reactivity with penicillin [87]. Despite this, the Joint Task Force on Practice Parameters; American Academy of Allergy, Asthma and Immunology; American College of Allergy, Asthma and Immunology; and Joint Council of Allergy, Asthma and Immunology [91] stated that "cephalosporin treatment of patients with a history of penicillin allergy, selecting out those with severe reaction histories, show a reaction rate of 0.1%." They recommend cephalosporin in cases without severe and/or recent penicillin-allergy reaction history when skin test is not available.

Macrolides, such as erythromycin and azithromycin, have limited efficacy against both *H. influenzae* and *S. pneumoniae* [69–72]. Clindamycin lacks efficacy against *H. influenzae*. Clindamycin alone (30–40 mg/kg per day in three divided doses) may be used for suspected PRSP; however, the drug will likely not be effective for the multidrug-resistant serotypes [69, 81, 88].

In the patient who is persistently vomiting or cannot otherwise tolerate oral medication, even when the taste is masked, ceftriaxone (50 mg/kg, administered intramuscularly in one or two sites in the anterior thigh, or intravenously) has been demonstrated to be effective for the initial or repeat antibiotic treatment of AOM [92, 93].

Although a single injection of ceftriaxone is approved by the US Food and Drug Administration (FDA) for the treatment of AOM, results of a double tympanocentesis study (before and 3 days after single-dose ceftriaxone) by Leibovitz et al. [93] suggest that more than one ceftriaxone dose may be required to prevent recurrence of the middle ear infection within 5–7 days after the initial dose.

Initial Antibiotic Treatment Failure

When antibiotics are prescribed for AOM, clinical improvement should be noted within 48–72 h. During the 24 h after the diagnosis of AOM, the child's symptoms may worsen slightly. In the next 24 h, the patient's symptoms should begin to improve. If initially febrile, the temperature should decline within 48–72 h. Irritability and fussiness should lessen or disappear, and sleeping and drinking patterns should normalize [94, 95]. If the patient is not improved by 48–72 h, another disease or concomitant viral infection may be present, or the causative bacteria may be resistant to the chosen therapy.

Some children with AOM and persistent symptoms after 48–72 h of initial antibacterial treatment may have combined bacterial and viral infection, which would explain the persistence of ongoing symptoms despite appropriate antibiotic therapy [96, 97]. Literature is conflicting on the correlation between clinical and bacteriologic outcomes. Some studies report good correlation ranging from 86 to 91 % [98, 99], suggesting continued presence of bacteria in the middle ear in a high proportion of cases with persistent symptoms. Others report that MEF from children with AOM in whom symptoms are persistent is sterile in 42–49 % of cases [100, 101]. A change in antibiotic may not be required in some children with mild persistent symptoms.

In children with persistent, severe symptoms of AOM and unimproved otologic findings after initial treatment, the clinician may consider changing the antibiotic. If the child was initially treated with amoxicillin and failed to improve, amoxicillin/clavulanate should be used. Patients who were given amoxicillin/clavulanate or oral third-generation cephalosporins may receive intramuscular ceftriaxone (50 mg/kg). In the treatment of AOM unresponsive to initial antibiotics, a 3-day course of ceftriaxone has been shown to be better than a 1-day regimen [93].

Although trimethoprim/sulfamethoxazole and erythromycin/sulfisoxazole had been useful as therapy for patients with AOM, pneumococcal surveillance studies have indicated that resistance to these two combination agents is substantial [69, 72, 102]. Therefore, when patients fail to improve while receiving amoxicillin, neither trimethoprimsulfamethoxazole [103] nor erythromycin/sulfisoxazole is appropriate therapy.

Tympanocentesis with culture of MEF should be considered for bacteriologic diagnosis and susceptibility testing when a series of antibiotic drugs have failed to improve the clinical condition. If tympanocentesis is not available, a course of clindamycin may be used, with or without an antibiotic that covers nontypeable *H. influenzae* and *M. catarrhalis*, such as cefdinir, cefixime, or cefuroxime.

Because *S. pneumoniae* serotype 19A is usually multidrug-resistant and may not be responsive to clindamycin [37, 72], newer antibiotics that are not approved by the FDA for treatment of AOM, such as levofloxacin or linezolid, may be indicated [104–106]. Levofloxacin is a quinolone antibiotic that is not approved by the FDA for use in children. Linezolid is effective against resistant Gram-positive bacteria. It is not approved by the FDA for AOM treatment and is expensive. In children with repeated treatment failures, every effort should be made for bacteriologic diagnosis by tympanocentesis with Gram stain, culture, and antibiotic susceptibility testing of the organism(s) present. The clinician may consider consulting with pediatric medical subspecialists, such as an otolaryngologist for possible tympanocentesis, drainage, and culture and an infectious disease expert, before use of unconventional drugs such as levofloxacin or linezolid.

When tympanocentesis is not available, a possible way to obtain information on the middle ear pathogens and their antimicrobial susceptibility is to obtain a nasopharyngeal specimen for bacterial culture. Almost all middle ear pathogens derive from the pathogens colonizing the nasopharynx, but not all nasopharyngeal pathogens enter the middle ear to cause AOM. The positive predictive value of nasopharyngeal culture during AOM (likelihood that bacteria cultured from the nasopharynx is the middle ear pathogen) ranges from 22 to 44 % for *S. pneumoniae*, 50–71 % for nontypeable *H. influenzae*, and 17–19 % for *M catarrhalis*. The negative predictive value (likelihood that bacteria not found in the nasopharynx are not AOM pathogens) ranges from 95 to 99 % for all three bacteria [107, 108]. Therefore, if nasopharyngeal culture is negative for specific bacteria, that organism is likely not the AOM pathogen. A negative culture for *S. pneumoniae*, for example, will help eliminate the concern for multidrug-resistant bacteria and the need for unconventional therapies, such as levofloxacin or linezolid. On the other hand, if *S. pneumoniae* is cultured from the nasopharynx, the antimicrobial susceptibility pattern can help guide treatment.

Duration of Therapy

The optimal duration of therapy for patients with AOM is uncertain; the usual 10-day course of therapy was derived from the duration of treatment of streptococcal pharyngotonsillitis. Several studies favor standard 10-day therapy over shorter courses for children younger than 2 years [84, 109–113]. Thus, for children younger than 2 years and children with severe symptoms, a standard 10-day course is recommended. A 7-day course of oral antibiotic appears to be equally effective in children 2–5 years of age with mild or moderate AOM. For children 6 years and older with mild to moderate symptoms, a 5–7-day course is adequate treatment.

Conclusion

The impact of AOM on child health far exceeds the discomfort and suffering associated with individual episodes of disease. AOM is among the largest drivers of antibiotic use in children. Providing support for prevention of the disease

is an important strategy for reducing antibiotic prescribing and subsequently the emergence of resistance. AOM and its treatment, and its complications, have a significant economic cost for the society.

References

1. Lieberthal AS, Carroll AE, Chonmaitree T, Ganiats TG, Hoberman A, Jackson MA, Joffe MD, Miller DT, Rosenfeld RM, Sevilla XD, Schwartz RH, Thomas PA, Tunkel DE. The diagnosis and management of acute otitis media. Pediatrics. 2013;131(3):964–99.
2. Chonmaitree T, Heikkinen T. Role of viruses in middle-ear disease. Ann N Y Acad Sci. 1997;830:143–57.
3. Klein JO, Bluestone CD. Otitis media. In: Feigin RD, Cherry JD, Demmler-Harrison GJ, Kaplan SL, editors. Textbook of pediatric infectious diseases. 6th ed. Philadelphia: Saunders; 2009. p. 216–37.
4. Chonmaitree T, Revai K, Grady JJ, et al. Viral upper respiratory tract infection and otitis media complication in young children. Clin Infect Dis. 2008;46(6):815–23.
5. Ruohola A, Meurman O, Nikkari S, et al. Microbiology of acute otitis media in children with tympanostomy tubes: prevalences of bacteria and viruses. Clin Infect Dis. 2006;43(11):1417–22.
6. Ruuskanen O, Arola M, Heikkinen T, Ziegler T. Viruses in acute otitis media: increasing evidence for clinical significance. Pediatr Infect Dis J. 1991;10(6):425–7.
7. Chonmaitree T. Viral and bacterial interaction in acute otitis media. Pediatr Infect Dis J. 2000;19(suppl 5):S24–30.
8. Nokso-Koivisto J, Räty R, Blomqvist S, et al. Presence of specific viruses in the middle ear fluids and respiratory secretions of young children with acute otitis media. J Med Virol. 2004;72(2):241–8.
9. Yano H, Okitsu N, Hori T, et al. Detection of respiratory viruses in nasopharyngeal secretions and middle ear fluid from children with acute otitis media. Acta Otolaryngol. 2009;129(1):19–24.
10. Grieves JL, Jurcisek JA, Quist B, et al. Mapping the anatomy of respiratory syncytial virus infection of the upper airways in chinchillas (*Chinchilla lanigera*). Comp Med. 2010;60:225–32.
11. Murphy TF, Chonmaitree T, Barenkamp S, Kyd J, Nokso-Koivisto J, Patel JA, Heikkinen T, Yamanaka N, Ogra P, Swords WE, Sih T, Pettigrew MM. Panel 5: microbiology and immunology panel. Otolaryngol Head Neck Surg. 2013;148:64–89.
12. Heikkinen T, Osterback R, Peltola V, Jartti T, Vainionpaa R. Human metapneumovirus infections in children. Emerg Infect Dis. 2008;14:101–6.
13. Martin ET, Fairchok MP, Kuypers J, et al. Frequent and pro- longed shedding of bocavirus in

young children attending day- care. J Infect Dis. 2010;201:1625–32.

14. Longtin J, Bastien M, Gilca R, et al. Human bocavirus infections in hospitalized children and adults. Emerg Infect Dis. 2008;14:217–21.

15. Beder LB, Hotomi M, Ogami M, et al. Clinical and microbiological impact of human bocavirus on children with acute otitis media. Eur J Pediatr. 2009;168:1365–72.

16. Rezes S, Soderlund-Venermo M, Roivainen M, et al. Human bocavirus and rhino-enteroviruses in childhood otitis media with effusion. J Clin Virol. 2009;46:234–7.

17. Savolainen-Kopra C, Blomqvist S, Kilpi T, Roivainen M, Hovi T. Novel species of human rhinoviruses in acute otitis media. Pediatr Infect Dis J. 2009;28:59–61.

18. Yano H, Okitsu N, Watanabe O, et al. Acute otitis media associated with cytomegalovirus infection in infants and children. Int J Pediatr Otorhinolaryngol. 2007;71:1443–7.

19. Ishizuka S, Yamaya M, Suzuki T, et al. Effects of rhinovirus infection on the adherence of *Streptococcus pneumoniae* to cultured human airway epithelial cells. J Infect Dis. 2003;188:1928–39.

20. Tuomanen EI. The biology of pneumococcal infection. Pediatr Res. 1997;42:253–8.

21. Cundell DR, Gerard NP, Gerard C, et al. *Streptococcus penumoniae* anchor to activated human cells by the receptor for platelet-activating factor. Nature. 1995;377:435–8.

22. Krishnamurthy A, McGrath J, Cripps AW, Kyd JM. The incidence of *Streptococcus pneumoniae* otitis media is affected by the polymicrobial environment particularly *Moraxella catarrhalis* in a mouse nasal colonisation model. Microbes Infect. 2009;11:545–53.

23. Moore HC, Jacoby P, Taylor A, et al. The interaction between respiratory viruses and pathogenic bacteria in the upper respiratory tract of asymptomatic Aboriginal and non-Aboriginal children. Pediatr Infect Dis J. 2010;29:540–5.

24. Tomochika K, Ichiyama T, Shimogori H, Sugahara K, Yamashita H, Furukawa S. Clinical characteristics of respiratory syncytial virus infection–associated acute otitis media. Pediatr Int. 2009;51:484–7.

25. McGillivary G, Mason KM, Jurcisek JA, Peeples ME, Bakaletz LO. Respiratory syncytial virus–induced dysregulation of expression of a mucosal beta-defensin augments colonization of the upper airway by non-typeable *Haemophilus influenzae*. Cell Microbiol. 2009;11:1399–408.

26. Bluestone CD, Klein JO. Microbiology. In: Bluestone CD, Klein JO, editors. Otitis media in infants and children. 4th ed. Hamilton: BC Decker; 2007. p. 101–26.

27. Del Beccaro MA, Mendelman PM, Inglis AF, et al. Bacteriology of acute otitis media: a new perspective. J Pediatr. 1992;120(1):81–4.

28. Block SL, Harrison CJ, Hedrick JA, et al. Penicillin-resistant Penicillin-resistant *Streptococcus pneumoniae* in acute otitis media: risk factors, susceptibility patterns and antimicrobial management. Pediatr Infect Dis J. 1995;14(9):751–9.

29. Rodriguez WJ, Schwartz RH. *Streptococcus pneumonia* causes otitis media with higher fever and more redness of tympanic membranes than *Haemophilus influenzae* or *Moraxella catarrhalis*. Pediatr Infect Dis J. 1999;18(10):942–4.

30. Pichichero ME, Casey JR. Evolving microbiology and molecular epidemiology of acute otitis media in the pneumococcal conjugate vaccine era. Pediatr Infect Dis J. 2007;26(suppl 10):S12–6.

31. Block SL, Hedrick J, Harrison CJ, et al. Community-wide vaccination with the heptavalent pneumococcal conjugate significantly alters the microbiology of acute otitis media. Pediatr Infect Dis J. 2004;23(9):829–33.

32. Casey JR, Adlowitz DG, Pichichero ME. New patterns in the otopathogens causing acute otitis media six to eight years after introduction of pneumococcal conjugate vaccine. Pediatr Infect Dis J. 2010;29(4):304–9.

33. Ongkasuwan J, Valdez TA, Hulten KG, Mason EO Jr, Kaplan SL. Pneumococcal mastoiditis in children and the emergence of multidrug-resistant serotype 19A isolates. Pediatrics. 2008; 122:34–9.

34. Xu Q, Pichichero ME, Casey JR, Zeng M. Novel type of *Streptococcus pneumoniae* causing multidrug-resistant acute otitis media in children. Emerg Infect Dis. 2009;15:547–51.

35. Dagan R, Givon-Lavi N, Leibovitz E, Greenberg D, Porat N. Introduction and proliferation of multidrug-resistant *Streptococcus pneumoniae* serotype 19A clones that cause acute otitis media in an unvaccinated population. J Infect Dis. 2009;199:776–85.

36. Dagan R, Klugman KP. Impact of conjugate pneumococcal vaccines on antibiotic resistance. Lancet Infect Dis. 2008;8:785–95.

37. Pichichero ME, Casey JR. Emergence of a multiresistant serotype 19A pneumococcal strain not included in the 7-valent conjugate vaccine as an otopathogen in children. JAMA. 2007;298(15):1772–8.

38. Grubb MS, Spaugh DC. Microbiology of acute otitis media, Puget Sound region, 2005–2009. Clin Pediatr (Phila). 2010;49(8):727–30.

39. Revai K, McCormick DP, Patel J, Grady JJ, Saeed K, Chonmaitree T. Effect of pneumococcal conjugate vaccine on nasopharyngeal bacterial colonization during acute otitis media. Pediatrics. 2006;117(5):1823–9.

40. Pettigrew MM, Gent JF, Revai K, Patel JA, Chonmaitree T. Microbial interactions during upper respiratory tract infections. Emerg Infect Dis. 2008;14(10):1584–91.

41. O'Brien KL, Millar EV, Zell ER, et al. Effect of pneumococcal conjugate vaccine on nasopharyngeal colonization among immunized and unimmunized

children in a community-randomized trial. J Infect Dis. 2007;196(8):1211–20.

42. Jacobs MR, Bajaksouzian S, Windau A, Good C. Continued emergence of nonvaccine serotypes of *Streptococcus pneumoniae* in Cleveland. Proceedings of the 49th Interscience Conference on Antimicrobial Agents and Chemotherapy; 2009; G1G1556.

43. Hoberman A, Paradise JL, Shaikh N, et al. Pneumococcal resistance and serotype 19A in Pittsburgh-area children with acute otitis media before and after introduction of 7-valent pneumococcal polysaccharide vaccine. Clin Pediatr (Phila). 2011;50(2):114–20.

44. Thomas JC, Figueira M, Fennie KP, et al. *Streptococcus pneumoniae* clonal complex 199: genetic diversity and tissuespecific virulence. PLoS One. 2011;6:e18649.

45. Centers for Disease Control and Prevention (CDC). Licensure of a 13-valent pneumococcal conjugate vaccine (PCV13) and recommendations for use among children—Advisory Committee on Immunization Practices (ACIP), 2010. MMWR Morb Mortal Wkly Rep. 2010;59(9):258–61.

46. Segal N, Givon-Lavi N, Leibovitz E, Yagupsky P, Leiberman A, Dagan R. Acute otitis media caused by *Streptococcus pyogenes* in children. Clin Infect Dis. 2005;41(1):35–41.

47. Luntz M, Brodsky A, Nusem S, et al. Acute mastoiditis—the antibiotic era: a multicenter study. Int J Pediatr Otorhinolaryngol. 2001;57(1):1–9.

48. Nielsen JC. Studies on the aetiology of acute otitis media. Copenhagen: Ejnar Mundsgaard Forlag; 1945.

49. McCormick DP, Lim-Melia E, Saeed K, Baldwin CD, Chonmaitree T. Otitis media: can clinical findings predict bacterial or viral etiology? Pediatr Infect Dis J. 2000;19(3):256–8.

50. Palmu AA, Herva E, Savolainen H, Karma P, Mäkelä PH, Kilpi TM. Association of clinical signs and symptoms with bacterial findings in acute otitis media. Clin Infect Dis. 2004;38(2):234–42.

51. McCormick DP, Chandler SM, Chonmaitree T. Laterality of acute otitis media: different clinical and microbiologic characteristics. Pediatr Infect Dis J. 2007;26(7):583–8.

52. Leibovitz E, Asher E, Piglansky L, et al. Is bilateral acute otitis media clinically different than unilateral acute otitis media? Pediatr Infect Dis J. 2007;26(7):589–92.

53. Leibovitz E, Satran R, Piglansky L, et al. Can acute otitis media caused by *Haemophilus influenzae* be distinguished from that caused by *Streptococcus pneumoniae*? Pediatr Infect Dis J. 2003;22(6):509–15.

54. Palmu AA, Kotikoski MJ, Kaijalainen TH, Puhakka HJ. Bacterial etiology of acute myringitis in children less than two years of age. Pediatr Infect Dis J. 2001;20(6):607–11.

55. Bodor FF. Systemic antibiotics for treatment of the conjunctivitis-otitis media syndrome. Pediatr Infect Dis J. 1989;8(5):287–90.

56. Bingen E, Cohen R, Jourenkova N, Gehanno P. Epidemiologic study of conjunctivitisotitis syndrome. Pediatr Infect Dis J. 2005;24(8):731–2.

57. Barkai G, Leibovitz E, Givon-Lavi N, Dagan R. Potential contribution by nontypable *Haemophilus influenzae* in protracted and recurrent acute otitis media. Pediatr Infect Dis J. 2009;28(6):466–71.

58. Doern GV, Jones RN, Pfaller MA, Kugler K. *Haemophilus influenzae* and *Moraxella catarrhalis* from patients with community acquired respiratory tract infections: antimicrobial susceptibility patterns from the SENTRY antimicrobial Surveillance Program (United States and Canada, 1997). Antimicrob Agents Chemother. 1999;43(2):385–9.

59. Klein JO. Microbiologic efficacy of antibacterial drugs for acute otitis media. Pediatr Infect Dis J. 1993;12(12):973–5.

60. Barnett ED, Klein JO. The problem of resistant bacteria for the management of acute otitis media. Pediatr Clin North Am. 1995;42(3):509–17.

61. Nussinovitch M, Yoeli R, Elishkevitz K, Varsano I. Acute mastoiditis in children: epidemiologic, clinical, microbiologic, and therapeutic aspects over past years. Clin Pediatr (Phila). 2004;43(3):261–7.

62. Roddy MG, Glazier SS, Agrawal D. Pediatric mastoiditis in the pneumococcal conjugate vaccine era: symptom duration guides empiric antimicrobial therapy. Pediatr Emerg Care. 2007;23(11):779–84.

63. Broides A, Dagan R, Greenberg D, Givon-Lavi N, Leibovitz E. Acute otitis media caused by *Moraxella catarrhalis*: epidemiologic and clinical characteristics. Clin Infect Dis. 2009;49:1641–7.

64. Ruohola A, Meurman O, Nikkari S, Skottman T, Heikkinen T, Ruuskanen O. The dynamics of bacteria in the middle ear during the course of acute otitis media with tympanostomy tube otorrhea. Pediatr Infect Dis J. 2007;26:892–6.

65. Aguilar L, Alvarado O, Soley C, Abdelnour A, Dagan R, Arguedas A. Microbiology of the middle ear fluid in Costa Rican children between 2002 and 2007. Int J Pediatr Otorhinolaryngol. 2009;73:1407–11.

66. Guevara S, Soley C, Arguedas A, Porat N, Dagan R. Seasonal distribution of otitis media pathogens among Costa Rican children. Pediatr Infect Dis J. 2008;27:12–6.

67. Lysenko ES, Lijek RS, Brown SP, Weiser JN. Within-host competition drives selection for the capsule virulence determinant of *Streptococcus pneumoniae*. Curr Biol. 2010;20:1222–6.

68. Howie VM, Ploussard JH. Efficacy of fixed combination antibiotics versus separate components in otitis media. Effectiveness of erythromycin estrolate, triple sulfonamide, ampicillin, erythromycin estolatetriple sulfonamide, and placebo in 280 patients with acute otitis media under two. and one-half years of age. Clin Pediatr (Phila). 1972;11(4):205–14.

69. Jacobs MR, Bajaksouzian S, Windau A, Good C. Continued emergence of nonvaccine serotypes of *Streptococcus pneumoniae* in Cleveland. Proceed-

ings of the 49th Interscience Conference on Antimicrobial Agents and Chemotherapy; 2009; G1G1556.

70. Tristram S, Jacobs MR, Appelbaum PC. Antimicrobial resistance in *Haemophilus influenzae*. Clin Microbiol Rev. 2007;20(2):368–89.

71. Critchley IA, Jacobs MR, Brown SD, Traczewski MM, Tillotson GS, Janjic N. Prevalence of serotype 19A *Streptococcus pneumoniae* among isolates from U.S. children in 2005–2006 and activity of faropenem. Antimicrob Agents Chemother. 2008;52(7): 2639–43.

72. Jacobs MR, Good CE, Windau AR, et al. Activity of ceftaroline against emerging serotypes of *Streptococcus pneumoniae*. Antimicrob Agents Chemother. 2010;54(6):2716–9.

73. Jacobs MR. Antimicrobial-resistant *Streptococcus pneumoniae*: trends and management. Expert Rev Anti Infect Ther. 2008;6(5):619–35.

74. Clinical and Laboratory Standards Institute. Performance standards for antimicrobial susceptibility testing: eighteenth informational supplement [document M100-S18]. Wayne: Clinical and Laboratory Standards, 2008.

75. Piglansky L, Leibovitz E, Raiz. S, et al. Bacteriologic and clinical efficacy of high dose amoxicillin for therapy of acute otitis media in children. Pediatr Infect Dis J. 2003;22(5):405–13.

76. Dagan R, Hoberman A, Johnson C, et al. Bacteriologic and clinical efficacy of high dose amoxicillin/clavulanate in children with acute otitis media. Pediatr Infect Dis J. 2001;20(9):829–37.

77. Hoberman A, Dagan R, Leibovitz E, et al. Large dosage amoxicillin/clavulanate, compared with azithromycin, for the treatment of bacterial acute otitis media in children. Pediatr Infect Dis J. 2005;24 (6):525–32.

78. Centers for Disease Control and Prevention (CDC). Licensure of a 13-valent pneumococcal conjugate vaccine (PCV13) and recommendations for use among children—Advisory Committee on Immunization Practices (ACIP), 2010. MMWR Morb Mortal Wkly Rep. 2010;59(9):258–61.

79. De Wals P, Erickson L, Poirier B, Pépin J, Pichichero ME. How to compare the efficacy of conjugate vaccines to prevent acute otitis media? Vaccine. 2009;27(21): 2877–83.

80. Shouval DS, Greenberg D, Givon-Lavi N, Porat N, Dagan R. Serotype coverage of invasive and mucosal pneumococcal disease in Israeli children younger than 3 years by various pneumococcal conjugate vaccines. Pediatr Infect Dis J. 2009;28(4): 277–82.

81. Harrison CJ, Woods C, Stout G, Martin B, Selvarangan R. Susceptibilities of *Haemophilus influenzae*, *Streptococcus pneumoniae*, including serotype 19A, and *Moraxella catarrhalis* paediatric isolates from 2005 to 2007 to commonly used antibiotics. J Antimicrob Chemother. 2009;63(3):511–9.

82. Siegel RM, Kiely M, Bien JP, et al. Treatment of otitis media with observation and a safety-net antibiotic prescription. Pediatrics. 2003;112(3 pt 1):527–531.

83. Nussinovitch M, Yoeli R, Elishkevitz K, Varsano I. Acute mastoiditis in children: epidemiologic, clinical, microbiologic, and therapeutic aspects over past years. Clin Pediatr (Phila). 2004;43(3):261–7.

84. Hoberman A, Paradise JL, Burch DJ, et al. Equivalent efficacy and reduced occurrence of diarrhea from a new formulation of amoxicillin/clavulanate potassium (Augmentin) for treatment of acute otitis media in children. Pediatr Infect Dis J. 1997;16(5):463–70.

85. Arguedas A, Dagan R, Leibovitz E, Hoberman A, Pichichero M, Paris M. A multicenter, open label, double tympanocentesis study of high dose cefdinir in children with acute otitis media at high risk of persistent or recurrent infection. Pediatr Infect Dis J. 2006;25(3):211–18.

86. Atanaskovi-Markovi M, Velickovi TC, Gavrovi-Jankulovi M, Vuckovi O, Nestorovi B. Immediate allergic reactions to cephalosporins and penicillins and their cross-reactivity in children. Pediatr Allergy Immunol. 2005;16(4):341–7.

87. Pichichero ME. Use of selected cephalosporins in penicillin-allergic patients: a paradigm shift. Diagn Microbiol Infect Dis. 2007;57(suppl 3):13S–8S.

88. Pichichero ME, Casey JR. Safe use of selected cephalosporins in penicillin-allergic patients: a meta-analysis. Otolaryngol Head Neck Surg. 2007;136(3):340–7.

89. DePestel DD, Benninger MS, Danziger L, et al. Cephalosporin use in treatment of patients with penicillin allergies. J Am Pharm Assoc (2003). 2008;48(4):530–40.

90. Fonacier L, Hirschberg R, Gerson S. Adverse drug reactions to a cephalosporins in hospitalized patients with a history of penicillin allergy. Allergy Asthma Proc. 2005;26(2):135–41.

91. Joint Task Force on Practice Parameters, American Academy of Allergy, Asthma and Immunology, American College of Allergy, Asthma and Immunology, Joint Council of Allergy, Asthma and Immunology. Drug allergy: an updated practice parameter. Ann Allergy Asthma Immunol. 2010;105(4):259–73.

92. Green SM, Rothrock SG. Single-dose intramuscular ceftriaxone for acute otitis media in children. Pediatrics. 1993;91(1):23–30.

93. Leibovitz E, Piglansky L, Raiz S, Press J, Leiberman A, Dagan R. Bacteriologic and clinical efficacy of one day vs. three day intramuscular ceftriaxone for treatment of nonresponsive acute otitis media in children. Pediatr Infect Dis J. 2000;19(11):1040–5.

94. Rosenfeld RM, Kay D. Natural history of untreated otitis media. Laryngoscope. 2003;113(10):1645–57.

95. Rosenfeld RM, Kay D. Natural history of untreated otitis media. In: Rosenfeld RM, Bluestone CD, eds. Evidence-based otitis media. 2nd ed. Hamilton: BC Decker; 2003. p. 180–98.

96. Chonmaitree T, Owen MJ, Howie VM. Respiratory viruses interfere with bacteriologic response to antibiotic in children with acute otitis media. J Infect Dis. 1990;162(2):546–9.

97. Arola M, Ziegler T, Ruuskanen O. Respiratory virus infection as a cause of prolonged symptoms in acute otitis media. J Pediatr. 1990;116(5):697–701.

98. Dagan R, Leibovitz E, Greenberg D, Yagupsky P, Fliss DM, Leiberman A. Early eradication of pathogens from middle ear fluid during antibiotic treatment of acute otitis media is associated with improved clinical outcome. Pediatr Infect Dis J. 1998;17(9):776–82.

99. Carlin SA, Marchant CD, Shurin PA, Johnson CE, Super DM, Rehmus JM. Host factors and early therapeutic response in acute otitis media. J Pediatr. 1991;118(2):178–83.

100. Casey JR, Pichichero ME. Changes in frequency and pathogens causing acute otitis media in 1995–2003. Pediatr Infect Dis J. 2004;23(9):824–8.

101. Teele DW, Pelton SI, Klein JO. Bacteriology of acute otitis media unresponsive to initial antimicrobial therapy. J Pediatr. 1981;98(4):537–9.

102. Doern GV, Pfaller MA, Kugler K, Freeman J, Jones RN. Prevalence of antimicrobial resistance among respiratory tract isolates of *Streptococcus pneumoniae* in North America: 1997 results from the SENTRY antimicrobial surveillance program. Clin Infect Dis. 1998;27(4):764–70.

103. Leiberman A, Leibovitz E, Piglansky L, et al. Bacteriologic and clinical efficacy of trimethoprim-sulfamethoxazole for treatment of acute otitis media. Pediatr Infect Dis J. 2001;20(3):260–4.

104. Humphrey WR, Shattuck MH, Zielinski RJ, et al. Pharmacokinetics and efficacy of linezolid in a gerbil model of *Streptococcus pneumoniae*-induced acute otitis media. Antimicrob Agents Chemother. 2003;47(4):1355–63.

105. Arguedas A, Dagan R, Pichichero M, et al. An open-label, double tympanocentesis study of levofloxacin therapy in children with, or at high risk for, recurrent or persistent acute otitis media. Pediatr Infect Dis J. 2006;25(12):1102–9.

106. Noel GJ, Blumer JL, Pichichero ME, et al. A randomized comparative study of levofloxacin versus amoxicillin/clavulanate for treatment of infants and young children with recurrent or persistent acute otitis media. Pediatr Infect Dis J. 2008;27(6): 483–9.

107. Howie VM, Ploussard JH. Simultaneous nasopharyngeal and middle ear exudate culture in otitis media. Pediatr Digest. 1971;13:31–5.

108. Gehanno P, Lenoir G, Barry B, Bons J, Boucot I, Berche P. Evaluation of nasopharyngeal cultures for bacteriologic assessment of acute otitis media in children. Pediatr Infect Dis J. 1996;15(4):329–2.

109. Cohen R, Levy C, Boucherat M, Langue J, de La Rocque F. A multicenter, randomized, double-blind trial of 5 versus 10 days of antibiotic therapy for acute otitis media in young children. J Pediatr. 1998;133(5):634–9.

110. Pessey JJ, Gehanno P, Thoroddsen E, et al. Short course therapy with cefuroxime axetil for acute otitis media: results of a randomized multicenter comparison with amoxicillin/clavulanate. Pediatr Infect Dis J. 1999;18(10):854–9.

111. Cohen R, Levy C, Boucherat M, et al. Five vs. ten days of antibiotic therapy for acute otitis media in young children. Pediatr Infect Dis J. 2000;19(5):458–63.

112. Pichichero ME, Marsocci SM, Murphy ML, Hoeger W, Francis AB, Green JL. A prospective observational study of 5-, 7-, and 10-day antibiotic treatment for acute otitis media. Otolaryngol Head Neck Surg. 2001;124(4):381–7.

113. Pessey JJ, Gehanno P, Thoroddsen E, et al. Short course therapy with cefuroxime axetil for acute otitis media: results of a randomized multicenter comparison with amoxicillin/clavulanate. Pediatr Infect Dis J. 1999;18(10):854–9.

Abnormal Innate and Adaptive Immunity in Otitis Media

Jizhen Lin

Otitis media (OM) is one of the most common diseases of childhood, accounting for frequent physician's office visits, tympanic membrane surgeries, and antimicrobial therapy in the USA [1]. OM is an infection frequently caused by polymicrobial agents, including upper respiratory predominant commensal bacteria (most commonly *Streptococcus pneumoniae*, nontypeable *Haemophilus influenzae*, and *Moraxella catarrhalis*) and common upper respiratory viruses (most commonly influenza A, respiratory syncytial virus, adenovirus, and rhinovirus) under the abnormal innate and adaptive immunity of the middle ear mucosa. This had not been recognized till recently when programmed death ligand 1 (PD-L1) was identified from the middle ear mucosa of human patients and animal inflamed bullae. It is not quite clear why the middle ear mucosal infection leads to such an adverse condition: immunosuppression of T cells. There are several aspects of immunity in this particular organ which need to be further studied in order to understand why common flora and resident respiratory viruses clone and grow easily in the middle ear cavity, instead of other organs.

First of all, the middle ear is located at the dead end of the upper respiratory tract. The Eustachian tube is open only when one swallows. Oxygen is relatively low in the middle ear cavity. Second, innate and adaptive immunity in the

middle ear is somehow weakened or ignored compared with other organs in the body. It has long been recognized that homograft replacement of the tympanic member survives without any immunosuppressive therapy postoperatively [2]. This suggests that the middle ear is tolerant to homograft tissues. The middle ear is, thus, considered an immune-privileged area, just like the eyes, a well-known case of immune-privileged concept. Third, cascade inflammatory and immune reactions in the middle ear are somewhat different from other organs in the body because of the above anatomy and immune tolerance status, that is, middle ear infection tends to have more chances to be chronic due to the difficulty in discharging inflammatory cells, secretion, and debris as well as incompetence to kill invading microorganisms in time. In an organ located at the dead end, it is not easy to discharge invading microorganisms. With the accumulation of debris and metabolites of microorganisms, the middle ear mucosa has a tendency to produce abundant inflammatory cytokines and mediators such as tumor necrotic factor alpha (TNF-α) and interferon gamma (IFN-γ).

It has long been recognized that abnormality of the Eustachian tube predisposes the middle ear to infectious diseases. Microorganisms including commensals or flora and overt pathogens grow and thrive when the Eustachian tube is blocked and the mucociliary blanket is impaired. Usually, the innate and adaptive immune systems function in fighting off invading microorganisms. Innate immunity in the Eustachian tube and middle ear includes: barrier functions (e.g., mucous membrane and mucociliary blanket), sensing

J. Lin (✉)
Department of Otolaryngology, University of Minnesota
Hospitals and Clinics, 2001 6th Street SE, Room 216,
LRB, Minneapolis, MN 55455, USA
e-mail: linxx004@umn.edu

© Springer International Publishing Switzerland 2015
D. Preciado (ed.), *Otitis Media: State of the art concepts and treatment*, DOI 10.1007/978-3-319-17888-2_6

of microorganism receptors such as toll-like receptors (TLRs) [3, 4] of the resident middle ear epithelial cells and special inflammatory and immune-response-relevant cells such as mucosal dendritic cells (DCs) and mast cells [5], release of antimicrobial peptides and proteins (e.g., defensins and lysozymes) [6, 7], and recruitment and activity of various effector cells (e.g., neutrophils, macrophages, fibroblasts, natural killer cells, eosinophils) [8].

It has been recently shown that the Id1 protein affects the innate immunity by inducing the expression of inflammatory cytokines (TNF-α, IFN-γ, and Interleukin-8, IL-8), increasing mucin glycoprotein production, and allowing for proliferation of the middle ear cells; all these processes ultimately drive the mucociliary blanket system [9–11]. Our recent findings indicate that specific mucins and mucin chaperones relevant to the mucociliary blanket are increased in OM with effusion [12, 13]. On the other hand, other cytokines and mediators such as TNF-α and IFN-γ related to the cellular immunity of the middle ear are essential for the defense against middle ear infection. It is not clear whether humoral immunity is involved in the predisposition for OM: Some investigators reported a decreased IgG antibody level in OM patients [14], and some did not.

Innate Immunity The innate immune system serves as a first line of defense against invading bacteria and viruses. It recognizes and responds to the invading microorganisms in a generic way. There are cellular and humoral components of the innate immune system which confer mucosal protection from infection. In the upper respiratory tract, the most noteworthy antibacterial substance is lysozyme, which is present in the mucus blanket and in middle ear effusion. In the humoral part of the innate immunity, the most important component is secretory IgA, a polymer consisting of six IgA monomers, trapping invading microorganisms in a nonspecific way. Defensins are also important for the innate immunity of the middle ear and Eustachian tube. Cellular components of the innate immunity include macrophages, which engulf the invading microorganisms, and neutrophils that are major infection fighters in killing

microorganisms. Basically, the above mentioned components of the innate immunity are upregulated in the middle ear mucosa and cavity under the condition of acute OM or OM with effusion.

Mucous Membranes The structural integrity of the upper respiratory tract, that is, the mucous membrane, forms an effective barrier to invading microorganisms. Respiratory flora is restricted from entry because of the mucous membrane. In OM with effusion, usually it is thickened in response to inflammation. Most infectious agents, however, impinge on the mucous membranes of the upper respiratory tract, and from these sites most infections occur. Damage to the epithelial cells caused by toxic products of these bacteria may play a role in susceptibility to further infection of the middle ear mucosa.

Mucociliary Clearance The passage of airway in the Eustachian tube is lined with mucociliary blanket, a moist lining of the airway respiratory epithelium and cilia immersed in a thin layer of mucus. On top of the thin layer of mucus is a second viscous layer of mucus in which foreign particles and microorganisms are trapped. Within the thin layer of mucus, the cilia act out movements coordinated in direction towards the nasopharynx. Thereby the viscous layer of mucus including its freight is transported off in direction towards the nasopharynx. In OM with effusion, it is often shown that the mucociliary clearance is impaired. Optimum functionality of mucociliary clearance is dependent upon the normal Eustachian tube functionality. Under the condition of OM with effusion, there is often obstruction of the Eustachian tube or functional impairment of the Eustachian tube.

Cellular Defense Neutrophils, macrophages, mast cells, and lymphocytes are involved in innate immunity. Neutrophils, macrophages, and mast cells are the ones mainly for inflammation whereas lymphocytes (B and T cells), accounting for antibody-mediated immunity and cell-mediated immunity, respectively, are the ones mainly for adaptive immune responses. Cells involved in the innate immune system are always present and ready to mobilize and fight invading microorganisms. Typical cellular components for the innate immunity are physical epithelial barriers, phagocytic leukocytes, DCs, and natural killer cells. On the other hand, components of the adaptive immune system are usually silent; however, when activated, these components adapt to the invading agents through antibodies produced by B cells and cell-mediated immunity by T cells. DCs, in the inner lining of Eustachian tube and middle ear, act as antigen-presenting cells (APCs), good at processing antigen material of invading microorganisms and then presenting it onto the cell surface of DCs for detection by T cells. DCs also migrate to the lymph nodes where they interact with T cells and B cells to prime them and initiate the process of T and B cell differentiation and maturation. Mucosal mast cells are rich in proteases, which contribute to innate immunity through releasing granules [15]. The origin of mucosal mast cells is from hematopoietic stem cells, and the proliferation of the latter is dependent on T cell cytokines [16] and stem cell factor [17] in the middle ear mucosa.

Definsins and Lysozymes Defensins bind to microbial antigens and adhesins, often attenuating toxic or inflammatory-inducing capacities. Binding is not generic; it appears to be both defensin specific and antigen specific. Binding of defensins to antigens may, in turn, alter the interaction of antigens with epithelial cells and APCs attenuating the production of proinflammatory cytokines. The binding of defensins to antigens may also facilitate the delivery of bound antigen to APCs in some cases via specific receptors. These interactions enhance the immunogenicity of the bound antigen in an adjuvant-like fashion.

Adaptive Immunity The adaptive immune system acts as a second line of defense. It is an antigen-based immune response. This process includes recruitment of infectious agent-specific lymphocytes, activation of T lymphocytes, and killing of infectious agents. Due to the multi-step process, the adaptive immune system requires some time to react to invading microorganisms. Usually, the nasopharynx, Eustachian tube, and

middle ear tolerate colonization by a flora that does no harm to the surrounding mucosa. It is common to see *S. pneumoniae* in the nasopharynx, Eustachian tube, and middle ear mucosa. If a microbe, such as *S. pneumonia*, grows in a large quantity and breaches the line of encirclement of the innate immunity, that is, there is loss of balance in the control between a host and microbe, it does not matter whether it is the normal flora or overt pathogen, an infection actually occurs. As a result, pathological harm to the nasopharyngeal, Eustachian tube, and middle ear mucosa is inevitable. In the middle ear, the mucosal layer is relatively thin compared with that in the nasopharynx, Eustachian tube, and the rest of the upper respiratory tract, allowing for further infection or the formation of biofilms. Biofilm is notorious for resisting to the adaptive and innate immune systems because of the dormancy of bacteria. Tendency of forming biofilm in the middle ear cavity indicates the abnormality of the innate immune system, unable to kill bacteria in time.

Different from the innate immunity, the antigen-based adaptive immune system exhibits an immunological memory. It acts to kill an invading organism when encountering it a second time.

Clearance of invading microorganisms requires cytotoxic CD8-positive T lymphocytes (CTLs) in the middle ear mucosa. The optimal activation of CTLs requires two signals. One is the interaction between T cell receptor (TCR) on the surface of a T cell and peptide-major histocompatibility complex (MHC) complex on the surface of an APC, typically DCs. The other is the interplay between costimulatory molecules such as CD28 of CTLs and CD80 of APCs. Among costimulatory molecules, there are several members in the family of B7/CD28. Some molecules in this family are capable of costimulating T cells such as CD28 whereas some molecules are capable of coinhibiting T cells such as PD-1. The former involves the activation of CTLs, and the latter involves the inhibition and exhaustion of CTLs, leading to the prolongation of chronic inflammation [18].

There is no evidence to indicate that OM patients have a systemic immune response issue. In response to the pathogen infection, the levels

Table 6.1 Immunoglobulin levels in MEF and serum from 30 acute OM patients

Samples	No. of sample	IgA	IgG	IgM
MEF	30	586.1±434.6	3033.8±1870.0	617.2±421.2
Serum	28	644.0±511.3	5948.0±3780.5	1241.5±910.9

Unit: μg/mL measured by radial immunodiffusion as described in referenced study
MEF middle ear fluid

of IgA and IgG in the serum and/or middle ear effusion of OM patients are basically higher compared with control [19–24]. However, some recurrent acute OM patients have an impaired humoral immune response to *S. pneumonia*. In this particular OM type, approximately 16.5 % of patients have defects in antibody-mediated immunity mainly with IgG2 deficiency, a main IgG responding to pneumococcal polysaccharides in adults [25–27]. However, IgG1, an immunoglobulin mainly responding to pneumococcal polysaccharides, is not reduced in children with recurrent OM. In any case, IgG2 switching to IgG1, for example, immunoglobulin class/isotype switching, is an important humoral biological mechanism that changes B cell production of antibody from one class to another, either from an isotype IgM to another isotype IgG or from a sub-isotype IgG1 to another sub-isotype IgG2. During this process, only the constant region portion of the antibody heavy chain changed but not the variable region of the heavy chain. However, many investigators indicate that the middle ear effusion has lower concentrations of IgG and IgM than serum. This is consistent with our data, in which immunoglobulins in the middle ear fluid (MEF) are lower than those in serum (Table 6.1). This suggests that middle ear mucosa is somehow immunosuppressive although it contains inflammatory cells and bacterial products which are stimulatory to the production of IgG, IgM, and IgA locally. However, normal middle ear mucosa does not contain IgG but IgA and IgM [5]. It is difficult to explain why the inflamed site in the middle ear cavity contains less IgG and IgM than serum if the production of immunoglobulins is not inhibited in the middle ear mucosa, in which there are a lot of infiltrated lymphocytes including B and T cells. Regarding the levels of IgG in the blood stream and middle ear effusion, there are no differences between OM patients and their controls [19–24].

Mucin Dysregulation in Middle Ear Mucosa Mucins are glycoproteins that are fairly important to the middle ear defense system, thought to be a part of the innate immune system. It was not recognized till recently that the knockout of the mucin gene Muc5b disturbs the function of the Eustachian tube and middle ear and causes acute and fulminant infectious OM [28]. It has been reported that MUC5B is the predominant mucin glycoprotein in chronic otitis media (COM) [29, 30].

Approximately 20 mucin genes have been identified so far. A total of 12 out of 20 mucins have been shown to be in the respiratory tract [12, 13]. However, three to four mucins are identified from the middle ear mucosa; they are MUC5AC, MUC5B, MUC4, and MUC1. Among them, MUC4 and MUC1 are basically membrane-bound mucins, not secretory ones, although they may appear in the middle ear effusion. Only MUC5B and MUC5AC are mucins found in COM [12, 30]. It is known that MUC5B in humans responds to chronic stimuli [30, 31]. Occasionally, MUC5AC may be upregulated in OM [30]. It is clear in the recent studies that MUC5B is the predominant one [12, 13, 29, 30, 32]. MUC5B is actually a mucin expressed in submucosal glands, instead of in the surface epithelia, but it is highly upregulated in COM [29, 31, 32].

It is not clear why MUC5B is highly upregulated, instead of MUC5AC. MUC5AC is expected to be upregulated because it is usually expressed in the epithelial cells including nasopharynx, Eustachian tube, and orifice of the Eustachian tube at the end of the middle ear. Gland-like structures are often observed in chronic OM patients [29, 31].

This observation has been confirmed by in situ hybridization, which shows clearly that MUC5AC positive mucous cells are dominant in the

Eustachian tube mucosa whereas MUC5B positive mucous cells are only in the mucous glands of the Eustachian tube and tracheal submucosal glands [12, 13, 31]. In the middle ear mucosa, few MUC5B messenger RNA (mRNA) transcripts are found in the biopsy specimens [29, 32].

These samples are free of COM because they have no history of OM. There are no inflammatory cells infiltrated when examined carefully. MUC5B mucin is a polymer, linked head-to-head. Under a microscope, mucous strings can be found [12, 13, 29, 32]. That is a molecular basis for trapping invading microorganisms.

Advances in Potential Bench to Bedside in OM Research

OM is basically an inflammatory disease. Recent studies indicate that there is an immune suppression issue on the basis of inflammation. The main reason is that some of the inflammatory cytokines and mediators such as IFN-γ and TNF-α are linked to immune responses in the human body. This implies that chronic OM frequently occurs probably due to the immunosuppression in the middle ear mucosa. It appears that Id1 is an important regulatory transcription factor in the regulation of OM propensity. Id1 is linked to the mucin expression in the middle ear epithelial cells, infiltration of δγ T cells in the middle ear mucosa, and the proliferation of the middle ear epithelial cells. These housekeeping roles of Id1 in the middle ear have been recognized in the recent years and play an important role in the innate and adaptive immunity of the middle ear. The essence of Id1 in the middle ear epithelial cells makes it indispensable in the defense of invading microorganisms. Without Id1, the middle ear develops naturally occurring OM with effusion due to weakened innate and adaptive immunity. With too much Id1, the middle ear runs into a status in which predisposition of OM prevails by increasing inflammatory cytokines and mediators.

In conclusion, advancing the immunological and inflammatory mechanisms of OM patho-physiology will go a long way towards developing novel molecular targeting therapeutic strategies for this condition.

References

1. Hoberman A, et al. Treatment of acute otitis media in children under 2 years of age. N Engl J Med. 2011;364(2):105–15.
2. Alford BR, McFarlane JR, Neely JG. Homograft replacement of the tympanic membrane. Laryngoscope. 1976;86(2):199–208.
3. Han F, et al. Role for Toll-like receptor 2 in the immune response to Streptococcus pneumoniae infection in mouse otitis media. Infect Immun. 2009;77(7):3100–8.
4. Komori M, et al. Pneumococcal peptidoglycan-polysaccharides regulate toll-like receptor 2 in the mouse middle ear epithelial cells. Pediatr Res. 2011;69(2):101–5.
5. Suenaga S, et al. Mucosal immunity of the middle ear: analysis at the single cell level. Laryngoscope. 2001;111(2):290–6.
6. Moon SK, et al. Effects of retinoic acid, triiodothyronine and hydrocortisone on mucin and lysozyme expression in cultured human middle ear epithelial cells. Acta Otolaryngol. 2000;120:944–9.
7. Kohlgraf KG, et al. Defensins as anti-inflammatory compounds and mucosal adjuvants. Future Microbiol. 2010;5(1):99–113.
8. Mogi G. Mucosal immunity of the middle ear. Acta Otolaryngol Suppl. 1984;414:127–30.
9. Lin J, et al. Recognition of gene expression patterns in the ear of rats with cDNA microarray. Hear Res. 2003;175:2–13.
10. Hamajima Y, Lin J. Establishment of a chronic otitis media with mucoid effusion in rats with Id1 bollar transfection followed by obstruction of Eustachian tube. submitted; 2003.
11. Hamajima Y, et al. Id1 induces epithelial cell hyperplasia in the middle ear of rats. The eighth international symposium on recent advances in otitis media. Fort Lauderdale, Florida, USA: BC Decker; 2003.
12. Lin J, et al. Mucin production and mucous cell metaplasia in otitis media. Int J Otolaryngol. 2012;2012:745325.
13. Nakamura Y, et al. The role of atoh1 in mucous cell metaplasia. Int J Otolaryngol. 2012;2012:438609.
14. Prellner K, Kalm O, Pedersen FK. Pneumococcal antibodies and complement during and after periods of recurrent otitis. Int J Pediatr Otorhinolaryngol. 1984;7(1):39–49..
15. Kambe N, et al. Development of both human connective tissue-type and mucosal-type mast cells in mice from hematopoietic stem cells with identical distribution pattern to human body. Blood. 2004;103(3):860–7.

16. Bhattacharyya SP, et al. Activated T lymphocytes induce degranulation and cytokine production by human mast cells following cell-to-cell contact. J Leukoc Biol. 1998;63(3):337–41.

17. Mori A, et al. Analysis of stem cell factor for mast cell proliferation in the human myometrium. Mol Hum Reprod. 1997;3(5):411–8.

18. Hofmeyer KA, Jeon H, Zang X. The PD-1/PD-L1 (B7-H1) pathway in chronic infection-induced cytotoxic T lymphocyte exhaustion. J Biomed Biotechnol. 2011;2011:451694.

19. Howie VM, Ploussard JH. Efficacy of fixed combination antibiotics versus separate components in otitis media. Effectiveness of erythromycin estrolate, triple sulfonamide, ampicillin, erythromycin estolate-triple sulfonamide, and placebo in 280 patients with acute otitis media under two and one-half years of age. Clin Pediatr (Phila). 1972;11(4):205–14.

20. Sorensen CH, Nielsen LK. Plasma IgG, IgG subclasses and acute-phase proteins in children with recurrent acute otitis media. Apmis. 1988;96(8):676–80.

21. Berman S, et al. Immunoglobulin G, total and subclass, in children with or without recurrent otitis media. J Pediatr. 1992;121(2):249–51.

22. Misbah SA, et al. Antipolysaccharide antibodies in 450 children with otitis media. Clin Exp Immunol. 1997;109(1):67–72.

23. Drake-Lee AB, Hughes RG, Dunn C. Serum IgA and IgG functional antibodies and their subclasses to *Streptococcus pneumoniae* capsular antigen found in two aged-matched cohorts of children with and without otitis media with effusion. Clin Otolaryngol Allied Sci. 2003;28(4):335–40.

24. Corscadden KJ, et al. High pneumococcal serotype specific IgG, IgG1 and IgG2 levels in serum and the middle ear of children with recurrent acute otitis media receiving ventilation tubes. Vaccine. 2013;31(10):1393–9.

25. Freijd A, Oxelius VA, and B. Rynnel-Dagoo, A prospective study demonstrating an association between plasma IgG2 concentrations and susceptibility to otitis media in children. Scand J Infect Dis. 1985;17(1):115–20.

26. Veenhoven R, et al. Immunoglobulins in otitis-prone children. Pediatr Res. 2004;55(1):159–62.

27. Aghamohammadi A, et al. Immunologic evaluation of patients with recurrent ear, nose, and throat infections. Am J Otolaryngol. 2008;29(6):385–92.

28. Roy S, et al. Phenotype detection in morphological mutant mice using deformation features. Med Image Comput Comput Assist Interv. 2013;16(3):437–44.

29. Lin J, et al. Characterization of mucins in human middle ear and eustachian tube. Am J Physiol Lung Cell Mol Physiol. 2001;280:L1157–67.

30. Preciado D, et al. MUC5B Is the predominant mucin glycoprotein in chronic otitis media fluid. Pediatr Res. 2010;68(3):231–6.

31. Kawano H, et al. Identification of MUC5B mucin gene in human middle ear with chronic otitis media. Laryngoscope. 2000;110:668–73.

32. Lin J, et al. Expression of mucins in mucoid otitis media. JARO. 2003;4:384–93.

Basic Science Concepts in Otitis Media Pathophysiology and Immunity: Role of Mucins and Inflammation

7

Stéphanie Val

Part I: The Innate Immunity in Otitis Media

The first line of defense against pathogens entering in the middle ear is innate immunity. It plays very diverse and important roles:

- Creating a physical and chemical barrier to pathogens: cellular barriers that are the epithelial surfaces and mucus layers on the top of epithelia
- Identifying pathogens with nonspecific receptors or sensing molecules
- Producing factors to activate inflammation, called pro-inflammatory mediators as cytokines and chemokines, to attract inflammatory cells
- Activate the process of adaptive immunity response by recruiting cells and presenting them antigens
- Kill pathogens and clean them from the tissue.

Several pathogens were identified in the middle ear of patients suffering from OM: diverse bacteria and viruses. Sometimes both at the same time have been found in middle ear effusions (MEEs) and seem to help each other [1]. Against these invaders, cellular and molecular barriers, recognition molecules and receptors, inflammatory

mediators, and inducible effectors of the epithelium constitute the innate immune mechanisms that protect the middle ear.

The First Line of Defense of the Innate Immunity: Cellular and Humoral Barriers

The very first lines of defenses of the innate immunity are physical and functional barriers. They are the epithelium of the middle ear and eventually the layer of mucoid gel on the top of it to protect the cells of the epithelium from the invasion by pathogens. The middle ear cavity of healthy patients does not contain liquid. Contrary to the airways, this line of defense has to be activated in the middle ear.

The Middle Ear Epithelium

The epithelium of the middle ear is mostly a single layer of cubical squamous cells. Some patches of the middle ear epithelium, and especially close to the Eustachian tube, gradually change in a pseudostratified columnar epithelium similar to the mucociliary epithelium of respiratory epithelia [2]. This epithelium is constituted of basal cells, goblet cells producing mucins, and other cells that can be ciliated or not. On top of these patches, mucus is present and protects these regions of the epithelium from the infection. The ciliated cells ensure the movement of the mucus in direction to the Eustachian tube orifice where

S. Val (✉)
Sheikh Zayed Institute, The Otologic Laboratory, Children's National Health System, Center for Genetic Medicine Research, 111 Michigan Avenue NW, Washington, DC 20010, USA

© Springer International Publishing Switzerland 2015
D. Preciado (ed.), *Otitis Media: State of the art concepts and treatment*, DOI 10.1007/978-3-319-17888-2_7

it is evacuated from the middle ear to the oral cavity.

Mucus glands, a normal feature of the Eustachian tube, can also be present in the middle ear of patients with OM. They constitute invaginations of the epithelium in the lamina propria, regions very rich in goblet cells that are able to produce large quantities of mucins. In healthy subjects that did not have prior disease of the middle ear, very few mucus glands are usually observed, whereas in subjects that had a history of OM events, these glands are more numerous [3]. This suggests that in the middle ear, mucus glands probably appear after several episodes of OM and then remain even after the disease is resolved. In patients with chronic suppurative otitis media (CSOM), the density of mucus glands is very high [4] and appears as a sequelae of CSOM [5]. Studies of the structure of mucus glands in the middle ear showed that the epithelium first invaginates at the location of high-density goblet cells and then different ramifications develop to lead to different structure types and sizes. Nevertheless, it was noticed that mucus glands of the middle ear can degenerate and lose their ability to produce mucins [3] likely because when OM resolves, the ear contains less factors sustaining inflammation and mucin production.

As explained before, the healthy middle ear epithelium contains few goblet cells that are concentrated in some patches of mucociliary epithelium mainly close to the Eustachian tube. But in the case of OM, the simple layer epithelium remodels into a pseudostratified epithelium. Several studies have demonstrated by histology techniques (Hematoxilyn and eosin staining on cuts of paraffin-embedded tissues) that the middle ear epithelium exhibits more secretory cells as well as ciliated cells in numerous parts of the middle ear epithelium [6–8]. Secretory cells are positive to periodic acid Schiff (PAS) staining detecting the presence of glycoconjugates, which are mainly in mucin proteins. Smirnova et al. [9] demonstrated that these mucins are secreted in the MEEs as they were PAS positive using a slot blot.

The Mucus in the Middle Ear: An Important Role for Mucins

OM is characterized by the presence of fluid in the middle ear cavity, called effusions that can be serous or mucous. Serous effusions do not contain mucins and are not viscous. On the contrary, mucous effusions are highly viscous and contain a high content of mucins [10]. An in vitro test of transportability of a bead under magnetic attraction also indicated that mucous effusions are less transportable than serous ones, suggesting that mucous effusions are difficult to clear in the middle ear [11]. Serous effusions contain proteins similar to the blood, so it is suggested that serous fluids are the result of a passive transudate of blood components in the middle ear due to a negative pressure in the middle ear likely because of the Eustachian blockade during inflammatory OM [12, 13]. Even if there are some conflicting findings from different research groups, serous effusions are believed to show better outcomes of the disease, whereas mucoid effusions are suggested to predict chronic otitis media with effusions (COME) [11, 14]. The study of Matkovic et al. [15] also contributed to this hypothesis as among 108 effusions collected, only 6% were mucoid for patients having OM diagnosed for less than 3 months, whereas 95% were mucoid for patients having the disease for more than 3 months. The large differences in medical outcomes and effusion and middle ear mucosa (MEM) characteristics prove that various cellular and molecular pathways act in the evolution of the disease. The production of large amounts of mucins necessitates the differentiation of goblet cells in the epithelium and the development of mucin glands. Indeed, the reabsorption of water in serous fluids and the concentration of their proteins are believed to participate to turning serous effusions into mucous ones [16]. Contrary to serous effusions, mucous effusion production necessitates the active process of producing mucins (exudates). But as a large number of proteins from the blood are also present in the mucous effusions (as albumin the predominant one), a passive diffusion of proteins and liquid is also probably implicated in the accumulation of mucous effusions.

Ion transport and water channels are also believed to play an important role in bringing water in the middle ear cavity and participate to serous and mucous effusion production. The healthy middle ear has to be kept without fluid contrary to the inner ear for a good transmission of the sound vibrations. Herman et al. [17] suggested the importance of water channels and ion transports. Experiments conducted in Mongolian gerbil's middle ear cells showed that the absorption of fluid in the middle ear was dependent on an osmotic gradient created by sodium and potassium adenylpyrophosphatase (ATPase)-dependent channels. The impairment of this ion flux has been shown in the lungs of rabbits in response to hydrogen peroxide that is produced during oxidative processes as well as hypoxia, a condition likely to appear in OM [18]. The aquaporins (AQP)1, 4, and 5, channels regulating the water homeostasis in cells, were detected in the Eustachian tube and MEM of rats as well as the epithelial sodium channels (ENaCs) [19]. In experimental OM in rats induced by Eustachian tube obstruction, ENaC and AQP were deregulated from 1 to 8 weeks after Eustachian tube obstruction, suggesting their implication in the water imbalance leading to fluid presence in the middle ear [20].

Effusions are composed of mucins but contain other proteins (antibacterial proteins, cytokines, etc.), lipids, deoxyribonucleic acid (DNA), and bacterial components [10, 14, 21], some of these substances being remains of dead bacteria and epithelial cells. Mucins, the major macromolecular component of epithelial mucus, are very high-molecular-weight proteins constituted of a backbone where numerous sugar side chains are added as a posttranslational modification (glycosylation with glycotransferases enzymes). These glycoconjugates are linked to the mucins in the Golgi and are then stored in secretory granules, waiting to have a signal to merge with the membrane and be released in the extracellular compartment [22]. Mucins are widely studied as their regulation is often a key determinant of diseases as cancer, lung diseases, and gastrointestinal diseases.

Mucins are classified by their protein backbone that is encoded by different mucin genes called MUC. MUC transcripts are big (until 15 kilo bases), so is the protein backbone, accounting for 15–50 % of mucin mass, and can contain 400 to more than 11,000 amino acids [22]. The major posttranslational modification of mucins is O-glycosylations, consisting in O-glycans attached to tandem repeats rich in serine and threonine all along the backbone. N-glycosylation is also observed but in a lesser extent. More than 20 human MUC genes have been identified—about the same number in mice. Considering the size of their gene transcript and protein backbone, but also their many glycoconjugates, the analysis of the MUC proteins is difficult. In the respiratory tract, 12 MUC genes have been identified and less in the ear, probably because mucins are more studied in the airways. Studies of mucins in the MEM and MEEs seem to show that MUC5B is the predominant mucin in the ear of patients having OM, whereas healthy subjects show very low levels of mucin [6–8, 23, 24]. But other mucins have been detected, apparently in lower amounts, which are MUC5AC, MUC2, and MUC4 [7, 13, 24, 25]. MUC5B has been detected by transcript analysis and protein assay: Preciado et al. [23] detected MUC5B protein by mass spectrometry in MEEs from COME patients and Lin et al. [7] by immunohistochemistry on the mucosa of patients with mucoid OM, whereas non-inflamed mucosa did not react with either of the antibodies anti-MUC5B and anti-MUC4. It has been noticed that the Eustachian tube of mucoid OM patients had MUC5B, MUC4, and also MUC5AC and MUC1 glycoproteins [8]. From the same study, electron microscopy of secretions from COME patients showed the presence of chain-like polymeric mucin. Some studies have detected the presence of messenger ribonucleic acid (mRNA) transcripts of MUC1, MUC2, MUC3, MUC4, MUC5AC, MUC5B, MUC7, MUC8, MUC9, MUC11, MUC13, MUC15, MUC16, MUC18, MUC19, and MUC20 [24–26], but gene expression does not always reflect the protein production and secretion. Indeed, Thornton et al. [27] showed that mucin gene expression in the airways was not always correlated to the presence of the protein. Mucins can be secreted or attached to the cell membrane. Among the mucins detected in the middle ear, we can notice that MUC5B and MUC5AC are secreted mucins, whereas MUC1 and MUC4 and are membrane-tethered mucins [22].

The overproduction of mucins leads to mucoid effusions that are hard to clear by the middle ear. Efforts have been made to try to prevent mucin overproduction, but a recent article pointed to the necessary presence of MUC5B in the innate immune response of airways and the ear. A study directed by Dr. Christopher Evans showed that the knockout of *Muc5b* in mice had a fast and dramatic effect on the mortality and morbidity due to infection of the airways leading to systemic infection [28]. Histology of the lungs showed an overproduction of *Muc5ac* probably to compensate the lack of *Muc5b,* but failed to protect the airways from infection. The ears were also infected by different bacteria and contained liquid as well as signs of inflammation. Thus, *Muc5b* glycoprotein is needed in the airways and the ear to protect mice against bacterial invasion and shows its central role in the innate immunity.

Antimicrobial Molecules in Effusions

MEEs contain other molecules that participate to the defense against pathogens. Antibacterial proteins efficiently kill bacteria and are very important in the innate immunity mechanisms. Defensins are broad-spectrum antimicrobial peptides, small (30–45 amino acids), rich in cationic amino acids, and stabilized by disulfide bounds that protect them from proteases [29]. Defensins have antimicrobial properties towards bacteria and viruses, are able to inhibit some bacteria toxins [30], and have pro-inflammatory activities stimulating cytokine and chemokine production [31]. Surprisingly, defensins have not been studied in patient samples, but in vivo and in vitro studies of experimental OM showed their induction in response to bacterial infection of the middle ear [32, 33]. Human β-defensin 2 (HBD2) was studied in vitro in order to determine the molecular pathways implicated in its induction. In human middle ear epithelial cells (HMEEsCs), HBD2 is under the control of the pro-inflamma-

tory cytokine interleukin (IL)1-β that activates Raf-MEK1/2 (mitogen-activated protein kinase kinase), the mitogen-activated protein kinase (MAPK) pathway [34]. *Non-typable Haemophilus influenzae (NTHi)* is also able to induce the expression of HBD2 first activating the toll-like receptor (TLR) 2 and then inducing protein 38 (p38) MAPK pathway [32]. HBD1 and HBD2 have also shown their ability to reduce *Streptococcus pneumonia (SP), Haemophilus influenzae (Hi),* and *Moraxella catarrhalis (MC)* growth in a liquid broth assay [35]. In Chinchilla, the orthologue of human β-defensin 3, chinchilla β-defensin 1, CBD1, had potent antimicrobial activity against *SP, Hi,* and *MC* [36]. Furthermore, chinchillas pretreated with recombinant CBD1 resulted in lower colonization of *NTHi* in the nasapharynx [37]. But bacteria are able to resist to defensins when they are growing in biofilms: Jones et al. [38] demonstrated that HBD3 binds to extracellular DNA constituting the matrix of *NTHi* biofilms, leading to the sequestration of HBD3 and thus diminishing the biological activity of an important defense of innate immunity.

Other antibacterial molecules are also part of the innate immune defense. Among them, the lysozyme is a cathelicidin (a cationic peptide) that has various effects, primarily damaging the membrane of bacteria. Lysozyme is present in MEEs of pediatric patients having OM, especially in mucous effusions compared to serous ones [12, 13, 39]. Giebink et al. [40] showed that the concentrations of lysozyme are more important in the MEEs of patients with COME positive for bacteria culture and suggested that this antibacterial agent was not only produced by polymorphonuclear leukocytes but also by the middle ear epithelium that accounted for 50–80 % of the lysozyme in the middle ear. Experimental OM in animals also demonstrated higher lysozyme detection in the middle ear: in response to *MC* in the Guiney pig [41] and in response to *SP* in chinchilla, this study also showed that more lysozyme were observed even when heat-killed bacteria were injected in the middle ear, suggesting that the production of lysozyme might be activated in response to membrane components of bacteria. Furthermore, mouse depleted of lysozyme also showed a higher susceptibility to OM development after *SP* infection [42], underlining the importance of lysozyme in the innate immune defense against bacteria.

Finally, some other antibacterial molecules poorly studied seem to play a role in the middle ear defense to pathogens: surfactant proteins as short palate, lung, and nasal epithelium clone (SPLUNC)-1, small cationic peptides, halocidin, and xylitol [29, 43].

Recognition of Pathogens

The System of the Complement

The complement system is a biochemical cascade composed of several peptides normally present as inactive forms. This system can be activated by different sequential cascades of enzymatic reactions in which proteins are sequentially cleaved and activated. The resulting effector molecules are C3a and C5a, also called anaphylatoxins. They are the most potent activation products of the complement that are able to induce a large diversity of effects as bacterial cytotoxicity, induction of pro-inflammatory cytokines production, and inflammatory cell activation [44]. The activation of the complement system depends on three pathways. The classical pathway consists in the recognition of immunoglobulin IgG and IgM complexes formed around pathogens that activate the C1 complex, activating C4 molecules to induce the activation of C3 and C5. The alternative pathway is triggered by carbohydrates, lipids, and proteins found on pathogens: C3 mediates the activation of the cascade. And the lectin pathway recognizes sugars at the microbial surface and leads to the activation of C4, C3, and finally C5.

Mediators of the complement activation have been found in MEEs and the MEM. Recently, He et al. [45] analyzed molecules of the component in effusions of children with recurrent OM by the enzyme-linked immunosorbent assay (ELISA). High amounts of C3a, C5a, and sC5-b9 were detected in the MEEs of patients having OM for more than 6 weeks. The concentration of C5a

was also strongly correlated to the concentration of IL-6 and IL-8 pro-inflammatory cytokines, suggesting a link between complement activation and the inflammatory effect they induce. Complement transcript induction was also observed in HMEEsCs in vitro in response to *SP* and *influenza A virus (IAV)*. Another study was conducted on effusions of patients with COME to assay the complement activation (C3a and C3 cleavage fragments) by ELISA and western blot analysis [46]. High concentrations of complement molecules were found and C3 activation was evaluated at 40 % of the total amount of C3 protein. They also noticed that C3a concentration was higher when effusions stayed longer in the ear and when children had multiple tube insertions, pointing C3a levels as a marker of the chronicity of OM. The complement activation leads to lysis of pathogens; this has been verified by Niarko-Markela and Meri [47] with erythrocytes of Guiney pigs exposed to MEEs from patients with otitis media with effusion (OME). Thirteen of the 38 MEEs tested had direct endogenous hemolytic activity, and 27 enhanced serum-initiated lysis. They also detected high levels of terminal complement complexes demonstrating the strong activation of the complement.

Receptors of the Innate Immunity

Multiple cell types and especially epithelial cells that are in contact with the external environment express innate immune receptors as Toll Like Receptors (TLRs). In the mucosal environment, mast cells and dendritic cells also express TLRs. The TLRs are pattern recognition receptors that recognize pathogen-associated molecular patterns (PAMPs). The activation of TLRs leads to the production of molecules also implicated in the innate immune response, as chemokines, cytokines, interferons (IFNs), and antimicrobial molecules described before. TLRs are type I transmembrane receptors with an extracellular N-terminal region with leucin-rich repeats and an intracellular toll-IL-1 receptor (TIR) domain. TLRs can form homodimers or heterodimers. The homodimers of TLR4, TLR5, TLR11, and the heterodimers of TLR2-TLR1 or TLR2-TLR6 bind to their respective ligands at the cell surface, whereas TLR3, TLR7-TLR8, TLR9, and TLR13 localize to the endosomes, where they sense microbial and host-derived nucleic acids. TLR4 localizes at both the plasma membrane and the endosomes. They each recognize specific types of PAMPs, for example, TLR1-TLR2 and TLR1-TLR6 recognize acylated peptides, TLR4 recognizes lipopolysaccharide (LPS), TLR3 targets double-stranded ribonucleic acid (RNA), and TLR9 recognizes bacterial DNA. TLR signaling is induced by their dimerization, dependent on ligand binding. All TLRs except TLR3 have a signaling pathway dependent on myeloid differentiation factor 88 (MyD88), activating the transcription factor NF-κB and then the expression of pro-inflammatory cytokines [48].

Several TLRs have been identified in the MEM and MEEs. TLR2, TLR4, TLR5, and TLR9 were found at the level of RNA and proteins in the MEM of both OM and non-OM patients [49]. For TLR2, TLR4, and TLR5, no difference of expression was found between non-OM and OM MEM, but their concentration was lower in the mucosa of patients with CSOM. In consequence, it was suggested that the clinical recovery of OM depends on TLR expression in the middle ear. There are conflicting evidences considering TLRs in MEEs and the correlation with the presence of bacteria. Lee et al. [50] observed effusions of patients with OME having lower TLR2, TLR6, and TLR9 mRNA when they are prone to have persistent OM and the level of TLRs is higher in culture-positive MEEs. Another study demonstrated the inverse for TLR9: less TLR9 mRNA is detected in culture-positive MEEs [51], whereas Lee et al. [52] failed to see any difference in TLR2, TLR4, TLR5, and TLR9 mRNA. Studying TLRs in MEEs might be accurate for assaying their presence in immune cells but does not take into account the epithelial cells playing an important role in the immune defense through TLRs. This might explain the differences described before. Nevertheless, animal studies showed that defects in TLR2 and TLR4 lead to the persistence of inflammation and mucosal metaplasia during OM [53].

Role of the Inflammation in OM

Inflammation is a central innate immune response activated by pro-inflammatory mediators (chemokines, cytokines) in order to attract and activate immune cells, stimulate the various innate immune defenses, and initiate the adaptive immune response to pathogens. This is a very efficient process involving different mediators and cells, but also deleterious if it does not resolve when the pathogens are no longer present. Inflammation is suspected to participate to the absence of resolution of OM especially in the case of COME and CSOM.

Pro-inflammatory Cytokines and Chemokines in OM

Pro-inflammatory cytokines and chemokines are characteristic of the inflammatory process: They are induced at early stages of the innate immune response until advanced stages to sustain the inflammation and to stimulate the adaptive immune response. Cytokines are usually associated to different types of immune response and can be produced by different cell types: epithelial cells, macrophages, neutrophils, dendritic cells, etc. Thus, cytokines that are known to play an important role in the innate immunity are tumor necrosis factor α (TNF-α), interleukins IL-1, IL-10, IL-12, IFNs, and chemokines like IL-8. The adaptive immunity is usually characterized by the cytokines IL-2, IL-4, IL-5, transforming growth factor β (TGF-β), IL-10, and IFN-γ production, TGF-β and IL-10 being able to repress inflammation. In addition, granulocyte-macrophage-colony-stimulating factor (GM-CSF) and granulocyte-colony-stimulating factor (G-CSF) are cytokines known to stimulate the differentiation of hematopoetic cells. Pro-inflammatory cytokines and chemokines have been detected many times in MEEs; the Table 7.1 summarizes some of the more recent studies assaying the content of cytokine protein in MEEs or MEM by ELISA or their transcripts by polymerase chain reaction (PCR) [15, 49, 50, 54–61]. Among the 11 studies listed, 12 different cytokines were detected in samples collected from children or adults with acute otitis media (AOM), OME, COME, and CSOM. Despite the fact that it is complicated to compare

Table 7.1 Pro-inflammatory mediator detection in middle ear effusions (MEEs) or middle ear mucosa (MEM) of patients with otitis media (OM)

Cytokine	Detected in	References
IL-8	36 MEEs, COME patients, 92%	[54]
–	108 MEEs, OM +/− 3 months, +	[15]
–	96 MEEs, OME, + (RNA)	[50]
–	46 MEEs, OME, +	[55]
IL-6	20 MEEs, AOM, +	[56]
–	96 MEEs, OME, + (RNA)	[50]
–	72 ears, MEM, COM/CSOM, + (RNA)	[49]
–	75 MEEs, OME persistent and/or recurrent, 83%	[57]
IL-12	96 MEEs, OME, + (RNA)	[50]
–	80 MEEs, OME adults, 100%	[58]
IL-1β	36 MEEs, COME patients, 67%	[54]
–	108 MEEs, OM +/− 3 months, +	[15]
–	30 MEEs children, 38 MEEs adults OM, +	[59]
–	72 ears, MEM, COM/CSOM, + (RNA)	[49]
–	75 MEEs, OME persistent and/or recurrent, 58%	[57]
IL-2	108 MEEs, OM +/− 3 months, +	[15]
–	80 MEEs, OME adults, 75%	[58]
IL-4	80 MEEs, OME adults, 41%	[58]
–	26 MEEs, OME, +	[60]
IL-5	80 MEEs, OME adults, 52%	[58]
–	26 MEEs, OME, +	[60]
TNF-α	36 MEEs, COME patients, 77%	[54]
–	108 MEEs, OM +/− 3 months, +	[15]
–	30 MEEs children, 38 MEEs adults OM, +	[59]
–	96 MEEs, OME, + (RNA)	[50]
–	72 ears, MEM, COM/CSOM, + (RNA)	[49]
–	75 MEEs, OME persistent and/or recurrent, 38%	[57]
IFN-δ	108 MEEs, OM +/− 3 months, +	[15]
–	96 MEEs, OME, + (RNA)	[50]
–	72 ears, MEM, COM/CSOM, + (RNA)	[49]
–	80 MEEs, OME adults, 83%	[58]
–	75 MEEs, OME persistent and/or recurrent, 51%	[57]
TGF-β	45 MEEs, adults, OME, +	[61]
IL-10	108 MEEs, OM +/− 3 months, +	[15]
–	96 MEEs, OME, + (RNA)	[50]
–	80 MEEs, OME adults, 18%	[58]
–	45 MEEs, adults, OME, +	[61]
TNF-β	36 MEEs, COME patients, 0%	[54]
–	108 MEEs, OM +/− 3 months, +	[15]

In the column "Detected in," the following information is given: number of MEEs or samples of MEM; type of OM detected; adult is specified—if nothing written, the samples come from children; % of samples positive for the analysis (+ means not specified in the study, assuming 100%)

OME otitis media with effusion, *AOM* acute otitis media, *COM* chronic otitis media, *COME* chronic otitis media with effusion, *CSOM* chronic suppurative otitis media, *RNA* ribonucleic acid

the quantity of cytokines in each study, it seems that IL-8, IL-6, IL-12, and IL-2 are detected in almost all the effusions. IL-1β, IL-4, IL-5, TNF-α, IFN-δ, TGF-β, and IL-10 were detected in less MEEs (40–80% for the studies detailing this parameter), and TNF-β showed conflicting evidences considering its presence. IL-8, IL-6, IL-12, IL-1β, TNF-α, IFN-δ, and IL-10 seem to be in higher concentrations in culture-positive samples and CSOM that are usually characterized by the presence of a strong bacterial infection. IL-8 and IL-10 were detected in higher concentrations in mucoid effusions compared to serous ones.

MEEs contain a variety of cytokines acting both in promoting inflammation and regulating the adaptive immune response. Some of them are produced in very high content especially when the bacterial infection persists. The chronic stages of OM also show a diversity of cytokines in high concentration in the middle ear, suggesting a persistence of inflammation in absence of pathogens. The Eustachian tube obstruction due to inflammation and the low transportability of mucoid effusions might limit the efficiency of the clearance of killed pathogens, letting PAMPs in the middle ear that still stimulate the immune responses, so do the cytokines in mucoid fluids that might accumulate without the possibility of being cleared from the middle ear. Some defects in cytokine production, dependent on genetic and environmental influence, might also explain why children tend to be prone to recurrent and persistent OM. Cytokines exhibit strong effects that, if not balanced, can lead to a disproportionate immune response. These cytokines are produced by epithelial cells but also immune cells. They are granulocytes as neutrophils, basophils, and eosinophils and phagocytic cells as macrophages and dendritic cells, all detected in MEEs of patients with OME [60, 62–64].

Innate Immunity to Adaptive Immunity in OM: Activation of Lymphocytes

As described before, several immunoregulator cytokines are present in MEEs of patients, underlining the importance of the role of the adaptive system in OM. They can be divided in two groups: TH1 and TH2 (meaning lymphocyte T helper). They represent the ability of lymphocytes T to differentiate in TH1 type, inducing cell-mediated immunity and inflammation, or TH2 that mediates the humoral immunity through the production of antibodies by differentiated lymphocytes B. The different cytokines detected in the MEEs show the activation of both pathways. CD4+ T

cells were detected in MEEs several times [9, 61], T cells that are naïve or differentiated. The lymphocyte subpopulation in MEEs was analyzed by flow cytometry in the study of Skotnicka et al. [65]. CD3+ T cells were dominating the population of lymphocytes, and the T helpers CD4+ were the majority. The ratio of CD4+/CD8+ cells was significantly higher in MEEs, but the proportion of CD8+ cells was lower in MEEs than in blood. These immune cells are suspected to come from adenoids in patients presenting this abnormality, as the population of lymphocytes of adenoids is important and similar to the middle ear [66]. Lymphocytes B have been identified in the middle ear as well. A study assayed the presence of lymphocytes in relation to the presence of antibodies against specific bacteria in 238 MEEs of patients with AOM [67]. The percentage of lymphocytes was higher in the ears with bacteria-specific antibodies than in the ears without, which correlated with a faster resolution of OM. The activation of the TH2-specific pathway inducing the differentiation of lymphocytes B to produce specific antibodies seem to also play an important role in the resolution of OM.

Part II: Molecular and Cellular Mechanisms Implicated in OM Pathogenesis

OM is a very common disease in children that sometimes evolves into chronic OM for reasons not yet understood. In order to prevent the evolution of the disease in a chronic stage that is difficult to treat, we need to understand the mechanisms implicated in OM development in response to bacteria, and how their interaction evolves into chronic OM. The innate immune system plays a central role in OM, so researchers investigated the different mechanisms implicated in its activation during the infection of the middle ear. In vivo and in vitro models were developed to better understand how the middle ear epithelium responds to bacteria, hoping to find new strategies to treat patients with OM.

In Vivo and In Vitro Models to Study OM Pathogenesis

Animal Models

Animals are useful models to investigate the cellular and molecular mechanisms implicated in OM. They permit to control the type of infection, the different stages of a disease, as well as the genetic background of the biological material. Comparing to in vitro studies, in vivo models allow taking into account the entire immune system and the interaction between different cell types being important in the resolution of infections. But we have to keep in mind that animal models have their limitations as their responses to pathogens might not be the same as the human ones, the differences being dependent on the species chosen. For the study of OM, rodents are widely used: chinchilla, mouse, rat, Guiney pig, and gerbil. According to the literature, mice and chinchillas are the main animals used in laboratories to study OM. Mouse is the first animal models used now as they are small, with a very controllable genetic background, easy to use in laboratories because a high diversity of reagents are compatible with this species. Nevertheless, mice have a very small middle ear, which is less convenient to induce OM by surgery as well as collecting MEEs. Chinchilla offers the possibility to have a bigger middle ear: the review of Ryan et al. [68] compared the middle ear volume observed in different studies. The average middle ear volume of the chinchilla is about 1.5 ml^3, whereas the one of a mouse is about 0.05 ml^3, so the middle ear volume of the chinchilla is 30 times bigger than the one of the mouse. It is consequently easier to manipulate the middle ear and recover MEEs that are sufficient in quantity to do several biological assays. The anatomy of the chinchilla ear has also been shown to be very close to the human one [69]; they do not often develop spontaneous OM [70], and they show similar responses to virus and bacteria in the course of OM compared to humans even if the pathogens colonizing humans are not usually the same as those of chinchillas (see [71]). Rats are also used in several studies and have the advantage of having a bigger middle

ear and more availability of reagents than chinchillas. Several interesting studies used rats to do a time course analysis of OM development.

OM is often induced by experimental obstruction of the Eustachian tube, leading to a negative pressure in the middle ear [72, 73]. Infection by bacteria can be coupled to this procedure to mimic better human OM. Bacterial injection can be made through the tympanic membrane but damaging this membrane lets other contaminants the possibility to enter in the middle ear. Injection via the ventral bulla is preferred as it does not damage the tympanic membrane and avoids contaminations. But it necessitates skills in microsurgery to avoid damaging the vessels and airways around the bulla. Infections post surgery can occur and may modify the immune response in the middle ear. Considering these limitations, Stol et al. [74] developed a noninvasive murine model adapted from a previous rat model. They used a pressure cabin at 40 kPa which induced *pneumococci* translocation from the nasopharyngeal cavity to the middle ear; the maximum bacteria load appearing 96 h post infection with the bacteria. Inflammation was confirmed with the secretion of IL-1β and TNF-α in the middle ear. This model has the advantage to avoid the limitations due to the surgery but probably does not permit to have homogenous OM development between animals. Another disadvantage should be considered: other parts of the body might be affected by the difference of pressure, especially for medium- or long-term experiments. Finally, pressure cabins might not be easy to use, expensive to buy, and might not permit to expose enough animals at the same time.

Human pathogens are studied in animal models as relevant clinical strains. But they are evolutionary adapted to humans and usually not animals, which can bring bias in these experimental studies. Nevertheless, the effects observed in experimental OM induced in animals and especially mice are very close to the observations made in humans: OM induced in mice having different genetic backgrounds with different strains of *SP, Hi,* and *MC* have shown similar inflammatory and mucosal effects even if the duration of the disease, the intensity of the responses, and the ability of resolution of OM where variable [68].

OM was also evaluated in mutant mouse strains; a strategy often used to investigate the implication of a specific gene in the apparition or the course of a disease. Mutations are natural or induced in laboratories. For the study of OM, we have to be careful choosing the type of mutations. Mutations in genes acting in the development of the middle ear might create some morphologic defects, influencing the responses of the middle ear. Mutating central genes in the immunity might also compromise the response to pathogens. And the deletion of a gene sharing similar functions with other genes sometimes leads to compensation mechanisms that may compensate the loss of functionality. Otherwise, this type of biological material offers great possibilities in studying spontaneous OM or pathogen-induced OM.

In Vitro Models

Transformed middle ear epithelial cells are now widely used to investigate the mechanisms implicated in bacteria effects, especially focusing on inflammatory and mucoid effects. This type of biological material permits to assay the effect of live bacteria, bacteria lysates, purified bacteria proteins, inflammatory mediators, etc., in a homogenous cell type which is useful but lacks the interaction with other cell types, especially the immune cells that produce mediators regulating epithelial cells. Knowing the limitations of cells in vitro, it is a very useful tool that gives us opportunities we cannot have with animals: the analysis of mechanisms implicated in a biological effect is more easy.

The human middle ear epithelial cell line HMEEC-1 was created by Dr. David Lim in 2002 using a retrovirus containing E6/E7 genes of human papillomavirus type 16 to transform primary middle ear epithelial cells from adults [75]. This type of transformation is known to regulate the cell cycle acting on the retinoblastoma (RB) tumor suppressor gene limiting the repression of the cell cycle and mediating the degradation of p53 protein also implicated in cell cycle repression [76, 77].

The mouse middle ear epithelial cell (mMEEsC) line was made by Dr. Jizhen Lin laboratory in 2005 [78]. Middle ear epithelial cells were isolated from mice and transformed by the large T-antigen of the simian virus 40 (SV40) A-gene. These cells have the property to be temperature sensitive: At 33 °C, the SV40 antigen is active and stimulates the cell cycle. But at 37/39 °C, SV40 is inactivated and cells differentiate, expressing markers of epithelial cells such as keratins and collagens. In our laboratory, we have noticed that these cells can be cultured several weeks at air liquid interface and form a single layer epithelium.

Other cell types were used: the middle ear cell line from chinchillas immortalized by SV40 [79] and the primary chinchilla middle ear epithelial cells (CMEEsCs) [80] or primary middle ear epithelial cells from adults successfully differentiated at air liquid interface in a ciliary and secretory epithelium [81]. Our laboratory tried to culture middle ear epithelial cells from children middle ear but because of the low amount of cells available during these procedures, we were unable to successfully grow them.

Interactions Between Pathogens and Ear Epithelial Cells

After having passed the eventual innate immune barriers in the middle ear, bacteria reach the middle ear epithelium. There, they adhere to the cells using adherence molecules varying depending on the bacteria. This part is focused on *NTHi* adhesion and invasion in airway and middle ear cells as *NTHi* is the main pathogen implicated in OM and as its interactions with epithelial cells has been widely studied.

NTHi is a gram-negative nonencapsulated bacterium that adheres and invades the middle ear. Several factors are necessary to its ability to invade epithelial cells. *NTHi* is able to secrete IgA proteases that increase its ability to adhere and invade the bronchial epithelial cells NCI-H292 [82]. Several factors produced by *NTHi* bind to host proteins: The protein F, a homolog of

SP lamin-binding proteins, is an adhesion factor that binds to the lamin of host cells [83]. Protein E has also been implicated in epithelial cell adhesion and the interaction with extracellular matrix proteins [84, 85]. Protein D, an outer membrane lipoprotein highly conserved, is important for *NTHi* adherence and is now used in *pneumococcal* polysaccharide conjugate vaccines that include monoacetylated protein D carriers, vaccines that showed their efficiency preventing OM development [86]. Finally, the phosphocholine (PCho) groups associated to the lipooligosaccharide of *NTHi* showed several times its implication in *NTHi* adherence as well as its ability to form biofilms [86–88]. PCho also present in *SP* was found to interact with the platelet-activating factor receptor (PAF receptor) as PAF present also PCho motifs recognized by this receptor [88]. In addition, the study of Van Schilfgaarde et al. [89] demonstrated that different clinical strains of *NTHi* elicited different patterns of adhesion, implying that some factors produced by specific strains might play a critical role in *NTHi* adhesion. They suggested that high molecular weight proteins are implicated in the virulence of the different clinical strains of *NTHi*.

NTHi has been detected on cells (adherence) and in cells (invasion). The presence of *NTHi* at the surface of epithelial cells was demonstrated by bacteria culture after infection [90], fluorescent microscopy techniques [89], and scanning electron microscopy, bacteria being mainly located on the top of non-ciliated cells [91]. Different molecular pathways in epithelial cells were found to play an important role in *NTHi* adhesion and invasion. The cytoskeleton with microtubules and actin were rearranged and necessary for *NTHi* virulence [90–92]. Macropinocytosis was demonstrated to be an important internalization mechanism of *NTHi* [91], and other studies found the implication of lipid rafts [92]. *NTHi* is also able to produce outer membrane vesicles that contain factors that will help the bacteria to invade hosts. These vesicles have a diameter of 20–200 nm and contain DNA, adhesins, and other enzymes [93]. These vesicles are internalized by caveolin-dependent mechanisms and

elicit the production of immune proteins as IL-8 and the antibacterial protein LL-37, surprisingly enhancing *NTHi* invasion in epithelial cells. Thus, different mechanisms are implicated in *NTHi* internalization in epithelial cells and might be dependent on cell culture conditions and the *NTHi* strain used.

In the middle ear, bacteria are found planktonic or organized in biofilms [94, 95]. The growth of bacteria in biofilms gives them the ability to hide from the immune system of the host and resist to antibiotics due to the extracellular matrix the bacteria create around them [95]. Biofilms of main pathogens in OM were detected in the middle ear of patients: *SP, Hi,* and *MC* but also *Staphylococcus aureus* and *Staphylococcus epidermidis*. But even if these bacteria are known to resist to high antibiotic quantities, we do not know yet how they can invade human cells. It is possible that biofilms are a defense mechanism to protect bacteria from a hostile inflammatory environment, offering them a niche to wait that immune responses decrease in order to better infect the host.

Regulation of Mucin Production and Mucous Cell Metaplasia in OM: Role of Pro-inflammatory Mediators

Inflammation and effusion production are characteristic of OM. As explained before, clinical inflammation seems to appear at the early stages of OM development when the middle ear tries to fight the infection by bacteria and/or viruses until more chronic stages even if the bacteria count seems lower. But this is not the case for mucin production that is mainly observed at later stages of OM course. Serous effusions are suspected to mainly come from the transudation of liquid and proteins from the blood, whereas mucous effusions need the active process of mucin production. Mucins are produced by goblet cells of the middle ear epithelium and mucus glands, which are easily detected in the MEM of patients with OME and COME, but at very low levels in healthy middle ears. These observations suggest that several factors play a role in the remodeling of the epithelium of the middle ear. This part of the chapter will try to review the different factors implicated in mucin production and mucous cell metaplasia, focusing on the inflammatory mediators that seem to play a crucial role in this process.

Infection of the Middle Ear by Bacteria Results in Pro-inflammatory Mediators Expression and Secretion In In Vivo And In Vitro Models

MEEs from patients with OM contain high concentrations of a panel of pro-inflammatory cytokines (see Sect. 3.3.1). In vivo studies were conducted to try to replicate the conditions of infection occurring in OM in order to analyze the expression and secretion of pro-inflammatory cytokines in the MEM and in MEEs mainly in mice, chinchillas, and rats (Table 7.1 and 7.2).

Several studies assayed the effect of live or killed *NTHi* or its purified endotoxins in the mouse middle ear (Table 7.2) [73, 96–98]. They used different protocols to induce OM (transtympanic injection of bacteria or bacterial components coupled to Eustachian tube obstruction in some cases), and all found similar pro-inflammatory cytokines to be induced in the middle ear at the level of RNAs or proteins (by PCR of the MEM or ELISA assay of MEEs). The cytokines TNF-α, IL-1α, IL-1β, IL-10, IL-6, MIP-2, KC, and IFN-δ were upregulated in response to *NTHi,* at various time points depending on the conditions of OM induction: from 6 h to 2 months post *NTHi* injection. Mac Arthur et al. [96] did a time course study of cytokine expression in the MEM. They found the mRNAs of *Mip-2, Il-6,* and *Kc* upregulated at all time points, but the fold inductions were higher at earlier times. Preciado et al. [97] confirmed this high early effect assaying *Mip-2* at day 1 and day 7 after *NTHi* lysates injection. *SP* was also used in other studies to induce OM. The different techniques used to induce *SP* infection (pressure cabin, intranasal exposure, or transtympanic injection) showed pro-inflammatory effects as well (IL-1α, IL-1β, TNF-α, MIP-2, IL-2, IL-6), effects occurring from 24 h to 15 days after *SP* exposure [74, 96, 99, 100].

Stol et al. [74] underlined the early effect on cytokine production in middle ear homogenates as IL-1β and TNF-α were induced at 48 and 96 h after nasopharyngeal infection by *SP* but not at 144 h. Endotoxins from *Salmonella Typhimurium* or LPS were used to induce OM in three studies by transtympanic inoculation [101–103]. All the cytokines cited before were also upregulated in these experiments, assaying the protein concentration in MEEs or middle ear washes. These inductions were observed at early stages (1 day post injection) until 3 days. This suggests that exposing the MEM to purified bacteria proteins induces AOM resolving with time as there are no live bacteria that sustain the innate immune response.

Fewer studies were conducted in chinchilla and rat species; some examples are listed in Table 7.3. These animals are bigger than mice and allow injecting bacteria directly in the bulla without drilling the tympanic membrane. In chinchilla, low or high quantity of live or killed *SP* was able to induce the secretion of IL-1β, IL-6, and TNF-α until 3 days after infection in MEEs in animals having previous Eustachian tube obstruction [72, 104]. In one of the studies, IL-1β was shown to be induced early (6 h post infection), whereas IL-6, IL-8, and TNF-α appeared later [104]. In rats, *SP* or nonviable *NTHi* were potent to induce all the panel of cytokines described before from 6 h to 7 days post infection [105, 106]. Different time-dependent expression profiles of pro-inflammatory cytokines are observed but seem to point TNF-α and IL-1β as early cytokines in the response to bacterial challenge, and they are sustained during the disease process. This is supported by human MEEs analysis [107], TNF-α being considered as a biomarker for OM with effusion persistence and chronicity [57, 108].

The importance of cytokines in the development of OM has been further investigated using mutant mice or wild-type mice treated with receptor antagonists or neutralization antibody. The use of an antagonist of IL-1 receptor during OM mediated by *Hi* in chinchilla showed better resolution of OM. In another study, mucous cell metaplasia induced in mouse in response to *NTHi* or *SP* was also shown to be less important

Table 7.2 Pro-inflammatory mediators detected in mouse models of otitis media (OM)

Reference	Bacterial species/ component	OM induction	Duration of infection	Cytokines deregulated (time point)	Technique
[98]	Heat killed *Hi*	TTI one ear, other ear not injected as control	6 h	TNF-α, IL-1α, IL-10, IL1β, IL-6, MIP-2, KC	Gene chip (mRNA) on MEM
[101]	LPS	TTI, saline as control	3, 6, 12, or 24 h	IL-1β, TNF-α, MIP-2, KC (24h, other ND); GM-CSF (6h)	ELISA of ME wash
[74]	*SP*	Pressure cabin, nasopharyngeal infection	48, 96, 144 h after nasopharyngeal infection	IL-1β, TNF-α (48hrs and 96hrs)	ELISA of MEH
[73]	*NTHi* purified endotoxins	ETO and then TTI, saline as control	3 days, 2 weeks, 2 months	TNF-α (3 time points), IL-1β (3 days), IFN-δ not consistent	ELISA of MEEs, in situ hybridization MEM
[99]	*SP* then *Influenza virus*	Intranasal exposure, saline as control	15 days after *SP* infection	IL-1α, pro-IL-1β, TNF-α, MIP-2	PCR (mRNA) of MEM
[97]	*NTHi* lysates	TTI, saline as control	1 day and 7 days	MIP-2 most induced gene	Microarray (mRNA)
[102]	endotoxins from *Salmonella typhimurium*	TTI, saline as control	6 h, 12 h, 1 day, 3 days, 7 days, and 14 days	IL-1α (up to 3 days), TNF-α (day 1 and 3)	ELISA of MEEs
[103]	endotoxins from *Salmonella typhimurium*	TTI, saline as control	24 h	MIP-2, IL-1β, IL-6	ELISA of ME wash
[100]	*SP*	TTI one ear, other ear not injected as control	24 h	TNF-α, IL-1β, IL2, IL-6	PCR (mRNA) of MEM
[96]	Heat killed *Hi*	TTI one ear, other ear not injected or saline	6, 24, 72 h, 1 week	MIP-2, IL-6, KC all time points but more at 6 h	PCR (mRNA) of MEM

Saline as control means the control group was injected with saline in the middle ear
TTI transtympanic injection, *ETO* Eustachian tube obstruction, *MEH* middle ear homogenate, *MEEs* middle ear effusions, *MEM* middle ear mucosa, *PCR* polymerase chain reaction, *ELISA* enzyme-linked immunosorbent assay, *LPS* lipopolysaccharide, *SP* Streptococcus pneumonia, *TNF* tumor necrosis factor, *IFN* interferon, *IL* interleukin, *GM-CSF* granulocyte-macrophage-colony-stimulating factor, *Hi* Haemophilus influenzae, *NTHi* non-typable Haemophilus influenzae, *KC* kinase C, *mRNA* messenger ribonucleic acid, *MIP* macrophage inflammatory protein, *ND* not determined

in IL-10 null mice [109]. These results implicate IL-1α, IL-1β, and IL-10 in the persistence of OM. IL-1β is produced as a pro-protein attached to the plasma membrane and requires cleavage to be secreted. The inflammasome, multiprotein complex implicated in the activation of inflammation is able to cleave the pro-IL-1β. A recent article evaluated the implication of the inflammasome, mutating its adaptor apoptosis-associated speck-like protein containing a CARD *(Asc)* in mice [110]. The inflammatory defects observed were linked to an increase in the degree and duration of mucosal epithelial hyperplasia in the middle ear of *Asc221-/-* mice as well as a delay in bacterial clearance. This shows that even if an overproduction of IL-1β tends to delay OM resolution, its absence or the absence of the inflammasome is deleterious.

HMEEsCs treated with bacterial components also exhibited an overexpression of cytokine genes as well as protein secretion [34, 111, 112], showing that the epithelial cells of the MEEs

Table 7.3 Pro-inflammatory mediators detected in chinchilla and rat models of OM

Reference	Animal species	Bacterial species/ component	OM induction	Duration of infection	Cytokines deregulated (time point)	Technique
[72]	Chinchilla	Heat killed SP	ETO and then injection superior bulla, saline as control	3 days after SP injection	IL-1β and TNF-α	ELISA of MEEs
[104]	Chinchilla	Low quantity SP	ETO and then injection superior bulla, saline as control	1–72 h	IL-1β, (6 h); IL-6, IL-8, TNF-α (72 h)	ELISA of MEEs
[105]	Rat	SP	ETO and 42 days after injection though bulla, saline as control	2 days and 7 days after SP	IL-1β, TNF-α, IL-6, IL-10, IL-8 in MEEs up to day 3. In MEM IL-1β same; IFN-δ, TNF-α W3/5 to W16; IL-6, IL-10, IL-8, TGF-β, MCP-1 biphasic	ELISA of MEEs and PCR on MEM (mRNA)
[106]	Rat	nonviable NTHi	Transbullar inoculation, saline as control	3, 6, 24, 48, 72 h after NTHi	In ME wash more IL-1β, IL-6, TNF-α (24 h, other time points ND), in MEM mRNA TNF-α (up to 6 h); IL-1α, IL-8 (up to 24 h); IL-1β, IL-6 (up to 48 h); IL-10 (up to 72 h)	ELISA of ME wash and PCR of MEM

Saline as control means the control group was injected with saline in the middle ear
ETO Eustachian tube obstruction, *ME wash* middle ear wash, *MEEs* middle ear effusions, *MEM* middle ear mucosa, *PCR* polymerase chain reaction, *ELISA* enzyme-linked immunosorbent assay, *SP* Streptococcus pneumonia, *TNF* tumor necrosis factor, *IL* interleukin, *NTHi* non-typable Haemophilus influenzae, *mRNA* messenger ribonucleic acid, *W* week, *MCP-1* Monocyte chemoattractant protein 1

alone are able to produce pro-inflammatory cytokines in response to bacteria exposure, the TLRs playing an important role in this effect [113, 114].

Infection of the Middle Ear by Bacteria Induces Mucin Production and Mucous Cell Metaplasia

Several laboratories have demonstrated that the infection of the middle ear of animals by *NTHi, SP* live or killed, or LPS results in middle ear mucous metaplasia similar to patient samples described in Sect. 2.1. In mice, the transtympanic injection of *NTHi* lysates or its purified endotoxins resulted in middle ear thickening and mucous cell metaplasia starting at day 3 after infection until 2 months [73, 97]. This was confirmed using rat models infected by *NTHi, SP,* or *MC* as rats inoculated with these bacteria developed high middle ear secretory capacity showing the presence of mucins by the detection of carbohydrates and a high goblet cell density with thickness of the MEEs [115–119]. After *NTHi, SP,* or *MC* infection, the middle ear goblet cell density reached a peak at 2 months after infection and remained until 6 months. Thus, the middle ear is subject to a gradual remodeling that can persist a long time after a single injection of bacteria. Hunter et al. [119] showed that 7 days after a single injection of LPS, rats with Eustachian tube obstruction developed middle ear goblet cell metaplasia and hyperplasia, but not the control group. These results underline the high responsiveness of the middle ear epithelium to a single injection of bacterial component when the Eustachian tube is obstructed.

In vitro experiments have been conducted to analyze the mucoid effect of live or lysed bacteria on HMEEsCs-1. The exposure to *NTHi, SP,* or *MC* revealed a potency of the HMEEsC-1 to activate the promoter of MUC5AC and the transcription of its mRNA [113, 120–125]. Coculture of HMEEC-1 with live *SP* also demonstrated an induction of MUC5AC mRNA and promoter [126]. Kerschner et al. [120] extended the study to other mucins in this cell type: they found mRNA induction of MUC5AC, MUC5B, and MUC2, this being more relevant with the clinical observations of mucins in the middle ear of patients with OM. None of these studies analyzed the mucin proteins. Importantly, mucins have more of a biological effect if they are secreted. It has been shown in airway cells that mucins can be stored in vesicles before being secreted [22], and as mentioned before, the activation of mucin genes does not always reflect the production of the protein [27]. The predominant mucin in the MEEs MUC5B is also very poorly studied and needs more attention in terms of its genetic regulation, as from it appears that MUC5AC plays less of an important role in OM. But MUC5B glycoprotein production in the middle ear is probably mainly dependent on mucus glands that are hard to model in vitro. A way to address this question would be to use a glandular model in three-dimensional (3D) gel as already described for human primary bronchial epithelial cells grown in a basement membrane matrix [127]. After 22 days of growth, the bronchial cells differentiated into glandular acini with a lumen and were able to secrete MUC5B in the lumen.

Inflammatory Mediators Regulate Mucin Production and Mucous Cell Metaplasia

Inflammation is activated very quickly after infection of the middle ear, whereas mucin production, dependent on mucous cell metaplasia, occurs later. The hypothesis suggested by several researchers is that inflammation drives mucous cell metaplasia in the middle ear during OM and in consequence increases the production of mucins in effusions. A simple way to address this question is to use animals exposed to a pro-inflammatory cytokine in the middle ear instead of bacterial components. A first experiment was done by Catanzaro et al. [128] in Guiney pigs. The animals were exposed to human recombinant IL-1, IL-2, or TNF-α injected through the tympanic membrane, and the ears were observed until 72 h post injection. IL-2 and TNF-α induced effusions in the ear that resolved at 48 h for TNF-α and 72 h for IL-2. IL-1 did not have any effect. The experiment was repeated in mice by Watanabe et al. [129] that injected IL-1β and compared it to *NTHi* LPS effect. Similar pathological changes were observed in the two groups compared to controls and showed an inhibition of effusion production in presence of IL-1 receptor antagonist. TNF-α effects were studied several times in rats: injection of TNF-α in the middle ear induced effusion production, subepithelial edema, neutrophil infiltration, and MUC2 mRNA in the MEM [130, 131]. Coupled with Eustachian tube obstruction, TNF-α injection stimulated mucous cell metaplasia and hyperplasia with abundant production of mucin glycoproteins [132]. IL-8 pro-inflammatory cytokine was also shown to induce the thickening of the middle ear epithelium and inflammatory cell infiltration in mice, effects comparable but stronger compared to heat-killed *SP* [133].

Similar experiments were conducted in vitro to analyze the effect of pro-inflammatory cytokine exposure on mucin expression in the middle ear epithelium. HMEEsC-1, normal MEEsC, or chinchilla MEEsC exposed to IL-1β or TNF-α showed an increase of mRNA production of MUC2, MUC5AC, MUC8, and/or MUC19 [80, 134, 135]. In addition, MUC19 mRNA was induced in HMEEsC-1 and chinchilla MEEsC in response to IL-6 and IL-8 [80]. The total mucin glycoprotein content, more relevant with the biological effect of mucins, was increased by the incubation of chinchilla MEEsC or HMEEsC-1 with IL-1β or TNF-α detected by PAS staining and scintillography technique [134, 136]. Nakamura et al. [137] analyzed the ability of middle ear epithelial cells to differentiate in goblet cells in vitro in response to TNF-α. He showed that the co-exposure of mMEEsC to TNF-α and retinoic acid differentiated the epithelial cells in mucus-like cells, whereas retinoic acid alone did not, demonstrating that TNF-α participates in mucous cell differentiation. Smirnova et al. [62] used a goblet cell type from the human colon, HT29-MTX cells, in order to assay the effect of IL-8 on cells already differentiated in mucin-producing cells. They demonstrated an increase of MUC5B and MUC5AC secretion in response to IL-8 in a dose- and time-dependent manner, which was sustained until 5 days.

These studies show that several cytokines including IL-1β and TNF-α induce middle ear metaplasia and hyperplasia as well as effusion production containing mucins in vivo. Further analyses in in vitro models of middle ear epithelium demonstrated that these cytokines induce mRNA expression of mucins, stimulate the secretion of mucins by goblet cells, and are able to participate to mucous cell differentiation. All together, these studies point pro-inflammatory cytokines as a key determinant in middle ear mucous cell metaplasia and mucin production in OM. The signaling pathways implicated in these effects will be developed in the next parts.

Role of the Innate Immune Receptors TLRs
As mentioned, TLR2, TLR4, TLR5, and TLR9 were found at the level of RNA and proteins in the MEM of both OM and non-OM patients [49]. The TLRs are receptors that recognize similar patterns in pathogens, they are the first sensors of infection in the middle ear. In animals, TLRs were demonstrated to play a critical role in OM. Mutant mice were used to investigate the impact of deficiencies in TLRs in OM. Mice mutated for TLR4, TLR2, or TLR9 showed a more profound and persistent inflammation with impaired bacterial clearance when infected by *NTHi* or *SP* [138–141]. The early TNF-α induction observed in wild-type mice was not occurring in TLR2-/- and TLR4-/- mice. Leichtle et al. [139] showed that TLR2-/- mice had a delayed IL-10 expression and a prolonged failure to clear bacteria, whereas TLR4-/- mice had only an early bacteria clearance impairment. TLR4-/- mice were also characterized by an absence of TLR2 induction, suggesting an involvement of TLR4 in TLR2 activation.

MyD88 and TRIF proteins, adaptors of TLRs that mediate parallel signaling pathways, were also mutated. MyD88 mediates IL-1β induction, whereas TRIF mediates IFN responses. TRIF-/- and MyD88-/- mice both showed a reduced but more persistent mucosal metaplasia and impairment to clear bacteria [142, 143]. If we compare the mucosal effects of these mutated mice to wild-type ones, we see that TLR2-/- mice as well as MyD88-/- mice have a sustained and higher thickening of the middle ear epithelium after *NTHi* inoculation in the ear compared to wild-type mice, whereas milder effects were observed for TLR4 or TRIF deficient mice [53].

The signaling pathways leading to pro-inflammatory mediators and mucin gene induction were studied in vitro, focusing on MUC5AC. Figure 7.1 shows a summary of *NTHi* effect on HMEEsC-1 and other cell types as airway cells, adapted from the results of five studies directed by Dr. Jian Dong Li [112, 114, 121, 122, 144]. *NTHi* seem to activate the TLR2 but not the TLR4 and require the mediators MyD88, interleukin-1 receptor-associated kinase 1 (IRAK), and TNF receptor-associated factor protein 6 (TRAF6) to activate p38 and nuclear factor κB (NF-κB) pathways, resulting in pro-inflammatory mediators and MUC5AC promoter activation and in consequence the initiation of their transcription. Other studies also implicated the central transcription factor in inflammation NF-κB in response to bacterial components or cigarette smoke in middle ear cells [145–147]. The protein kinase C (PKC) pathway activates CARD-containing MAGUK protein 1 (CARMA-1) that seems to be implicated in inflammasome assembly [148], and extracellular signal-regulated kinase (ERK) was also implicated in *NTHi* effects as well as the Tβ receptors (TβR) that dimerizes in response to *NTHi* and activates Smad3/Smad4 to induce MUC2. The outer membrane protein (OMP)-6 of *NTHi* demonstrated its ability to induce several biomarkers of these pathways, suggesting the high importance of this protein in *NTHi* biological effects in middle ear epithelial cells.

Interestingly, *SP* infection revealed different responses. Figure 7.2 summarizes the results of four studies on the mechanisms of MUC5AC in-

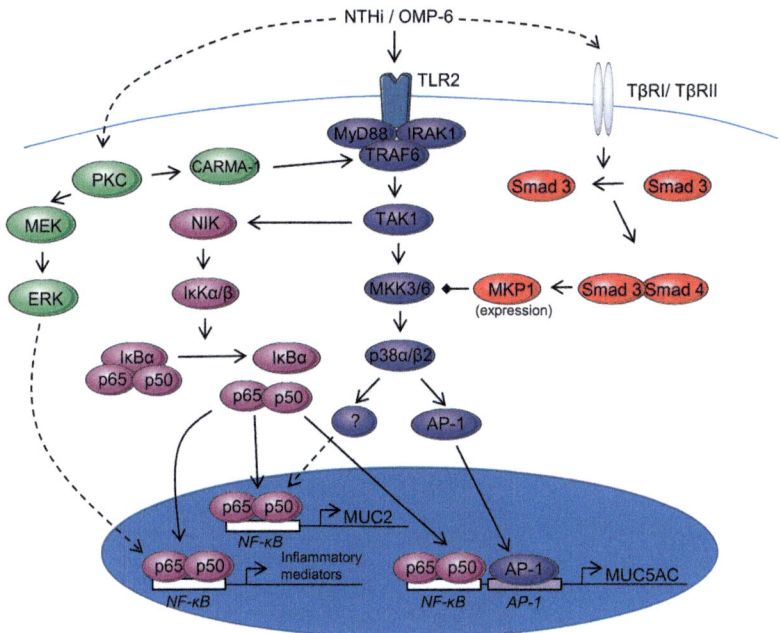

Fig. 7.1 Molecular pathways implicated in *non-typable Haemophilus influenzae (NTHi)* inflammatory and mucoid effects in human ear and airway epithelial cells. Four main molecular pathways have been identified in response to *NTHi* or its outer membrane protein *(OMP)-6:*1. Toll-like receptor 2 *(TLR2)* activates myeloid differentiation factor 88 *(MyD88)*, interleukin-1 receptor-associated kinase 1 *(IRAK1)*, TNF receptor-associated factor protein 6 *(TRAF6)*, TGF-β-activated kinase *(TAK1)*, MAP kinase kinase 3/6 *(MKK3/6)*, p38, activator protein 1 *(AP-1)* leading to MUC5AC and MUC2 transcription activation.2. *TAK1* induces a parallel signaling pathway activating NF-κB-inducing kinase *(NIK)*, IκKα/β (inhibitory IκB kinase), IκB phosphorylation detaching from p65/p50 that translocates to the nucleus to activate the transcription of MUC5AC and MUC2.3. TβRI/TβRII dimerization is induced by *NTHi*. It activates Smad3 that binds to Smad4 and induces the expression of MAP kinase phosphatase 1 *(MKP1)* inhibiting *MKK3/6* activation.4. *NTHi* activates protein kinase C *(PKC)* that activates CARD-containing MAGUK protein 1 *(CARMA-1)*, inducing TRAF6 signaling pathway. *PKC* also activates MAPK/ERK kinase *(MEK)* and then extracellular signal-regulated kinase *(ERK)* leading to the increase of p65/p50 binding to inflammatory mediator promoters.(Based on [112, 114, 121, 122, 144])

duction in response to *SP* lysates [113, 125, 126, 149]. Contrary to *NTHi, SP* activated TLR4 and not the TLR2 pathway. Nevertheless, the mediators MyD88, IRAK1, and TRAF6 were also implicated in TLR4 effects. Inhibitory IκB kinase (IκKα/β) was shown to be phosphorylated, leading to ERK activation by IκKα and repression by IκKβ. ERK activation resulted in MUC5AC transcription probably via the activator protein 1 (AP-1) factors. Jun kinase (JNK) was also activated in response to *SP* via TRAF6/p21-activated kinase 4 (PAK4), repressing the activation of MUC5AC. The protein MAP kinase phosphatase 1 (MKP1) was also demonstrated to repress ERK and JNK activation, conferring to the epithelial

cells the ability to limit MUC5AC induction in response to *SP* via different signaling pathways.

In consequence, from our knowledge TLRs especially TLR2 and TLR4 play an important role in the innate immune response to *NTHi* and *SP*. These receptors activate a quick inflammatory response to attract immune cells and clear pathogens. They regulate the production of pro-inflammatory mediators as well as mucin genes (MUC2 and MUC5AC). MUC5B is the predominant mucin in the MEEs of patients with OM; thus, it is important to further investigate the mechanisms of its regulation as well. TLR mutations in mice demonstrated a persistence of the middle ear metaplasia and hyperplasia, underlining the importance of its activation in the in-

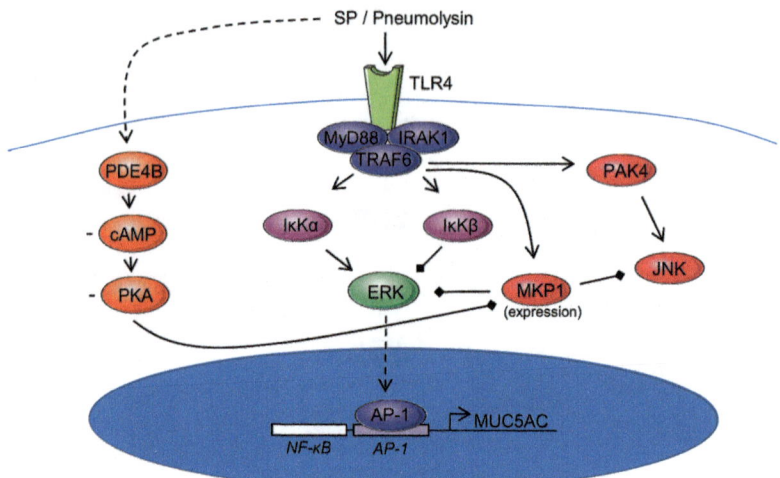

Fig. 7.2 Molecular pathways implicated in *Streptococcus pneumoniae (SP)* mucoid effects in human ear and airway cells. *SP* or its membrane protein pneumolysin activates three main signaling pathways:1. Toll-like receptor 4 *(TLR4)* activates myeloid differentiation factor 88 *(MyD88)*, interleukin-1 receptor-associated kinase 1 *(IRAK1)*, TNF receptor-associated factor protein 6 *(TRAF6)*, inhibitory IκB kinase *(IκKα/β)* that activates or represses extracellular signal-regulated kinase *(ERK)* leading to activator protein 1 *(AP-1)* translocation to the nucleus to bind to its responsive element in MUC5AC promoter and activate its transcription.2. *TRAF6* activates p21-activated kinase 4 *(PAK4)* and Jun kinase *(JNK)*. *TRAF6* also induces the expression of MAP kinase phosphatase 1 *(MKP1)* that represses *JNK* and *ERK*.3. *SP* also activates phosphodiesterase 4B *(PDE4B)* that reduces cyclic adenosine monophosphate *(cAMP)* content leading to less activation of protein kinase A *(PKA)* and the repression of *MKP1* expression.(Based on [113, 125, 126, 149])

flammatory responses during bacterial infection. Nevertheless, after the immune system resolved the bacterial infection, the inflammation has to stop. If it persists, it is likely that the middle ear epithelium remodels and exhibits a high number of goblet cells producing an excess of mucins.

Role of Hypoxia Mechanisms

Hypoxia is defined as an insufficient level of O_2 in the blood or a tissue. It induces responses of stress from cells trying to reduce their metabolism to save O_2 and try at the same time to bring more of it. The biomarkers of hypoxia are usually the transcription factor hypoxia inducible factor 1α (HIF-1α) and the secreted protein vascular endothelial growth factor (VEGF). During OM, the orifice of the Eustachian tube is often blocked, likely leading to a mild hypoxia in the middle ear. To investigate this direction, Sekiyama et al. [55] assayed the presence of VEGF in MEEs from patients with OME. VEGF was detected in high concentrations in MEEs and was associated to IL-8 secretion as well as endotoxins presence.

In vivo, the hypothesis that hypoxia regulates the responses observed during OM is supported by the fact that Eustachian tube obstruction induces MEEs and mucosal metaplasia [150]. This is also supported by the clinical observations of the Eustachian tube blockade during OM, due to inflammation, which stimulates the mucosal metaplasia of the middle ear [151]. A lower oxygenation of the middle ear can be a cause of hypoxia but the presence of a large amount of inflammatory cells during OM might participate to the consumption of O_2 as well. Kitaoka et al. [152] have also shown that *SP* consumes oxygen too, altogether the different cells (human cells and bacteria) additional to the Eustachian tube dysfunction are the cause of hypoxia.

Hypoxia induces stress responses dependent on oxygen radicals called reactive oxygen species as they react with the components of the cells (protein, lipids, DNA…) and damage them.

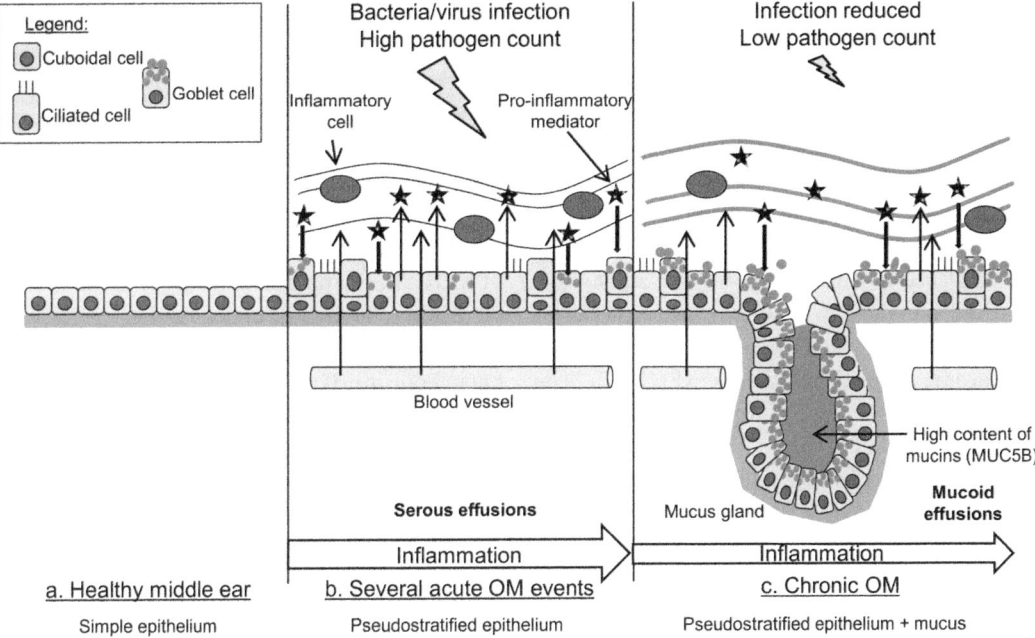

Fig. 7.3 Model suggested for the development of otitis media *(OM)* and the evolution into COME. **a** The healthy middle ear is represented in the part **a** as a single epithelium. The infection by bacteria induces inflammatory cytokine secretion in the middle ear which attracts inflammatory cells. **b** During middle ear inflammation, the Eustachian tube likely blocks and generates a negative pressure in the middle ear, leading to liquid and protein transudation from the blood, bringing liquid in the middle ear cavity. The pro-inflammatory mediators stimulate the middle ear epithelium to differentiate goblet cells. **c** In chronic stages of the disease, fewer bacteria are present in the middle ear. But the sustained inflammation remodeled the epithelium that has mucus glands producing large amounts of mucins, making the MEEs very viscous

High levels of lipid peroxidation, induced by an overproduction of reactive oxygen species, have been detected in MEEs of patients with OME [153, 154]. Balikci et al. [155] also showed evidence of protein oxidation in MEEs of patients with COME.

In vivo, rats with Eustachian tube blockade showed OM development and elevated expression of HIF-1α, VEGF, IL-1β, and TNF-α [156]. Two mutated mice were also characterized by the overexpression of the same hypoxia and inflammatory mediators: Jeff and Junbo mice [157]. Both mice having different mutations developed spontaneously OM and showed low O_2 levels in the middle ear and fluids as well as apoptotic polymorphonuclear inflammatory cells. The Junbo mice treated with an inhibitor of VEGF were seen to develop less hearing problems and mucosal metaplasia. The hypoxia was resolved by myringotomy of Junbo mice and associated with a reduction of the inflammation and the thickness of the MEM [158], showing the beneficial effect of middle ear oxygenation. The mechanisms under these effects were investigated with in vitro models grown in hypoxic conditions. Primary airway cells grown at 1% O_2 at air-liquid interface showed a dramatic differentiation in goblet cells positive for MUC5AC as well as a pseudostratified appearance and reduction of ciliated cells [159]. In another study, a bronchial cell line was demonstrated to secrete MUC5AC if cultured in hypoxic conditions, induction dependent on HIF-1α and Smad activation [160].

Hypoxia seems to participate in OM development, likely occurring during the inflammatory response of the middle ear epithelium. In addition to the innate immune response activated by pathogens, the increase in oxygen consumption in the middle ear coupled with the Eustachian tube obstruction might create a hypoxic environment. This can lead to the production of reactive oxygen species, creating some damages in the MEM, leading to the sustainment of inflammation.

In summary, from what we can summarize from the literature, we can suggest a model of OM development from very early responses to the chronic stage of the disease (Fig. 7.3). The healthy middle ear is a simple-layer epithelium (Fig. 7.3a) that keeps the middle ear without fluid which is assured by ion pumps and AQP water channels. When AOM events occur (Fig. 7.3b), the epithelial cells recognize pathogens with receptors which leads to the secretion of pro-inflammatory mediators. These mediators attract inflammatory cells (also producing pro-inflammatory mediators) and stimulate the remodeling of the epithelium, showing more cells producing mucins but also some ciliated cells. One of the consequences of the inflammation is to block the Eustachian tube thus impairing its function of clearance. A negative pressure in the middle ear likely occurs and induces the transudation of proteins and liquid from the blood. In addition, the impairment of ion pumps and water channels fail to reabsorb the water, letting serous fluids in the middle ear cavity. The infection can be managed by the immune system and the inflammation resolve, stopping the OM. If the inflammation persists, sometimes even in absence of pathogens or a low amount of bacteria as it has been described for COME, a more drastic remodeling of the middle ear epithelium occurs, leading to the production of more goblet cells as well as mucus glands that produce very large amounts of mucins (Fig. 7.3c). Proteins and water still diffuse from the blood vessels and participate in the production of a very viscous fluid due to the high content in mucins, mainly MUC5B.

Knowledge of mechanisms implicated in OM has increased dramatically over the past 20 years with new laboratory techniques for MEEs analysis, the use of mutant animals and in vitro models of middle ear epithelium. Nowadays, antibiotics are widely used but are not necessarily needed in certain cases like COME, where the bacteria infection has already been identified and treated by the innate immune system. Thus, efforts are needed to better understand what happens in the different stages of the disease to better guide patient treatment. This includes the study of MUC5B, the predominant mucin in MEEs, as there is a total lack of understanding of its regulation in OM. The recent study showing that the knoockout in MUC5B gene induces middle ear infection underlines this need [28]. The development of mucus glands probably produces a large amount of MUC5B present in MEEs. Their differentiation and regulation should also be addressed in OM with innovative cell culture strategies.

References

1. Marom T, Nokso-Koivisto J, Chonmaitree T. Viral-bacterial interactions in acute otitis media. Curr Allergy Asthma Rep. 2012;12(6):551–8.
2. Sade J. Middle ear mucosa. Arch Otolaryngol. 1966;84(2):37–43.
3. Tos M, Caye-Thomasen P. Mucous glands in the middle ear—what is known and what is not. ORL J Otorhinolaryngol Relat Spec. 2002;64(2):86–94.
4. Tos M, Bak-Pedersen K. Density of mucous glands in a biopsy material of chronic secretory otitis media. Acta Otolaryngol. 1973;75(1):55–60.
5. Tos M, Bak-Pedersen K. Density of mucous glands in various sequelae to otitis media. J Laryngol Otol. 1973;87(12):1183–92.
6. Kawano H, et al. Identification of MUC5B mucin gene in human middle ear with chronic otitis media. Laryngoscope. 2000;110(4):668–73.
7. Lin J, et al. Expression of mucins in mucoid otitis media. J Assoc Res Otolaryngol. 2003;4(3):384–93.
8. Lin J, et al. Characterization of mucins in human middle ear and Eustachian tube. Am J Physiol Lung Cell Mol Physiol. 2001;280(6):L1157–67.
9. Smirnova MG, Birchall JP, Pearson JP. Evidence of T-helper cell 2 cytokine regulation of chronic otitis media with effusion. Acta Otolaryngol. 2005;125(10):1043–50.
10. Carrie S, et al. Otitis media with effusion: components which contribute to the viscous properties. Acta Otolaryngol. 1992;112(3):504–11.
11. Dodson KM, Cohen RS, Rubin BK. Middle ear fluid characteristics in pediatric otitis media with effusion. Int J Pediatr Otorhinolaryngol. 2012;76(12):1806–9.

12. Yabe R, et al. Gel chromatographic characterization of proteins in mucous and serous middle ear effusions of patients with otitis media in comparison to serum proteins. Eur Arch Otorhinolaryngol. 2008;265(3):293–8.

13. Chung MH, et al. Compositional difference in middle ear effusion: mucous versus serous. Laryngoscope. 2002;112(1):152–5.

14. Kubba H, Pearson JP, Birchall JP. The aetiology of otitis media with effusion: a review. Clin Otolaryngol Allied Sci. 2000;25(3):181–94.

15. Matkovic S, Vojvodic D, Baljosevic I. Cytokine levels in groups of patients with different duration of chronic secretory otitis. Eur Arch Otorhinolaryngol. 2007;264(11):1283–7.

16. Tonder O, Gundersen T. Nature of the fluid in serous otitis media. Arch Otolaryngol. 1971;93(5):473–8.

17. Herman P, et al. Ion transport by primary cultures of Mongolian gerbil middle ear epithelium. Am J Physiol. 1992;262(3 Pt 2):F373–80.

18. Tate RM, et al. Oxygen-radical-mediated permeability edema and vasoconstriction in isolated perfused rabbit lungs. Am Rev Respir Dis. 1982;126(5):802–6.

19. Kang SH, et al. Expression of water channel proteins (aquaporins) in the rat Eustachian tube and middle ear mucosa. Acta Otolaryngol. 2007;127(7):687–92.

20. Song JJ, et al. Mucosal expression of ENaC and AQP in experimental otitis media induced by Eustachian tube obstruction. Int J Pediatr Otorhinolaryngol. 2009;73(11):1589–93.

21. FitzGerald JE, et al. Characterization of human middle ear mucus glycoprotein in chronic secretory otitis media (CSOM). Clin Chim Acta. 1987;169(2–3):281–97.

22. Rose MC, Voynow JA. Respiratory tract mucin genes and mucin glycoproteins in health and disease. Physiol Rev. 2006;86(1):245–78.

23. Preciado D, et al. MUC5B Is the predominant mucin glycoprotein in chronic otitis media fluid. Pediatr Res. 2010;68(3):231–6.

24. Elsheikh MN, Mahfouz ME. Up-regulation of MUC5AC and MUC5B mucin genes in nasopharyngeal respiratory mucosa and selective up-regulation of MUC5B in middle ear in pediatric otitis media with effusion. Laryngoscope. 2006;116(3):365–9.

25. Ubell ML, et al. MUC2 expression in human middle ear epithelium of patients with otitis media. Arch Otolaryngol Head Neck Surg. 2008;134(1):39–44.

26. Kerschner JE. Mucin gene expression in human middle ear epithelium. Laryngoscope. 2007;117(9):1666–76.

27. Thornton DJ, et al. Respiratory mucins: identification of core proteins and glycoforms. Biochem J. 1996;316(3):967–75.

28. Roy MG, et al. Muc5b is required for airway defence. Nature. 2014;505(7483):412–6.

29. Underwood M, Bakaletz L. Innate immunity and the role of defensins in otitis media. Curr Allergy Asthma Rep. 2011;11(6):499–507.

30. Lehrer RI, et al. Human alpha-defensins inhibit hemolysis mediated by cholesterol-dependent cytolysins. Infect Immun. 2009;77(9):4028–40.

31. Yang D, et al. Defensin participation in innate and adaptive immunity. Curr Pharm Des. 2007;13(30):3131–9.

32. Lee HY, et al. Induction of beta defensin 2 by NTHi requires TLR2 mediated MyD88 and IRAK-TRAF6-p38MAPK signaling pathway in human middle ear epithelial cells. BMC Infect Dis. 2008;8:87.

33. McGillivary G, et al. A member of the cathelicidin family of antimicrobial peptides is produced in the upper airway of the chinchilla and its mRNA expression is altered by common viral and bacterial co-pathogens of otitis media. Mol Immunol. 2007;44(9):2446–58.

34. Moon SK, et al. Synergistic effect of interleukin 1 alpha on nontypeable Haemophilus influenzae-induced up-regulation of human beta-defensin 2 in middle ear epithelial cells. BMC Infect Dis. 2006;6:12.

35. Lee HY, et al. Antimicrobial activity of innate immune molecules against Streptococcus pneumoniae, Moraxella catarrhalis and nontypeable Haemophilus influenzae. BMC Infect Dis. 2004;4:12.

36. Harris RH, et al. Identification and characterization of a mucosal antimicrobial peptide expressed by the chinchilla (Chinchilla lanigera) airway. J Biol Chem. 2004;279(19):20250–6.

37. McGillivary G, et al. Respiratory syncytial virus-induced dysregulation of expression of a mucosal beta-defensin augments colonization of the upper airway by non-typeable Haemophilus influenzae. Cell Microbiol. 2009;11(9):1399–408.

38. Jones EA, McGillivary G, Bakaletz LO. Extracellular DNA within a nontypeable Haemophilus influenzae-induced biofilm binds human beta defensin-3 and reduces its antimicrobial activity. J Innate Immun. 2013;5(1):24–38.

39. Harada T, Juhn SK, Adams GL. Lysozyme levels in middle ear effusion and serum in otitis media. Arch Otolaryngol Head Neck Surg. 1990;116(1):54–6.

40. Giebink GS, et al. Bacterial and polymorphonuclear leukocyte contribution to middle ear inflammation in chronic otitis media with effusion. Ann Otol Rhinol Laryngol. 1985;94(4 Pt 1):398–402.

41. Sato K. Experimental otitis media induced by nonviable Moraxella catarrhalis in the guinea pig model. Auris Nasus Larynx. 1997;24(3):233–8.

42. Shimada J, et al. Lysozyme M deficiency leads to an increased susceptibility to Streptococcus pneumoniae-induced otitis media. BMC Infect Dis. 2008;8:134.

43. Caye-Thomasen P, et al. Panel 3: Recent advances in anatomy, pathology, and cell biology in relation to otitis media pathogenesis. Otolaryngol Head Neck Surg. 2013;148(Suppl 4):E37–51.

44. M, P.P.a.K. Inflammation, Chronic Diseases and Cancer—Cell and Molecular. Biology, Immunology and Clinical Bases, D.M.K, editor, editor 2012.

http://www.intechopen.com/books/inflammation-chronic-diseases-and-cancer-cell-and-molec-ular-biology-immunology-and-clinical-bases/complement-receptors-in-inflammation. Accessed 17th April, 2015.

45. He Y, et al. Complement activation in pediatric patients with recurrent acute otitis media. Int J Pediatr Otorhinolaryngol. 2013;77(6):911–7.

46. Narkio-Makela M, Teppo AM, Meri S. Complement C3 cleavage and cytokines interleukin-1beta and tumor necrosis factor-alpha in otitis media with effusion. Laryngoscope. 2000;110(10 Pt 1):1745–9.

47. Narkio-Makela M, Meri S. Cytolytic complement activity in otitis media with effusion. Clin Exp Immunol. 2001;124(3):369–76.

48. O'Neill LA, Golenbock D, Bowie AG. The history of Toll-like receptors—redefining innate immunity. Nat Rev Immunol. 2013;13(6):453–60.

49. Si Y, et al. Attenuated TLRs in middle ear mucosa contributes to susceptibility of chronic suppurative otitis media. Hum Immunol. 2014;75(8):771–6.

50. Lee HY, et al. Toll-like receptors, cytokines & nitric oxide synthase in patients with otitis media with effusion. Indian J Med Res. 2013;138(4):523–30.

51. Lee HY, et al. Decreased expression of TLR-9 and cytokines in the presence of bacteria in patients with otitis media with effusion. Clin Exp Otorhinolaryngol. 2013;6(4):195–200.

52. Lee SY, et al. Clinical approaches for understanding the expression levels of pattern recognition receptors in otitis media with effusion. Clin Exp Otorhinolaryngol. 2011;4(4):163–7.

53. Leichtle A, et al. Innate signaling in otitis media: pathogenesis and recovery. Curr Allergy Asthma Rep. 2011;11(1):78–84.

54. Maxwell KS, et al. Interleukin-8 expression in otitis media. Laryngoscope. 1994;104(8 Pt 1):989–95.

55. Sekiyama K, et al. The role of vascular endothelial growth factor in pediatric otitis media with effusion. Auris Nasus Larynx. 2011;38(3):319–24.

56. Barzilaia A, et al. Middle ear effusion IL-6 concentration in bacterial and non-bacterial acute otitis media. Acta Paediatr. 2000;89(9):1068–71.

57. Yellon RF. et al. Cytokines, immunoglobulins, and bacterial pathogens in middle ear effusions. Arch Otolaryngol Head Neck Surg. 1995;121(8):865–9.

58. Kariya S, et al. TH1/TH2 and regulatory cytokines in adults with otitis media with effusion. Otol Neurotol. 2006;27(8):1089–93.

59. Park SN, et al. Expression of HSP70 and its relation with other cytokines in human middle ear effusion. Clin Exp Otorhinolaryngol. 2010;3(1):18–23.

60. Sobol SE, et al. T(H)2 cytokine expression in atopic children with otitis media with effusion. J Allergy Clin Immunol. 2002;110(1):125–30.

61. Zhao SQ, et al. Role of interleukin-10 and transforming growth factor beta 1 in otitis media with effusion. Chin Med J (Engl). 2009;122(18):2149–54.

62. Smirnova MG, Birchall JP, Pearson JP. In vitro study of IL-8 and goblet cells: possible role of IL-8 in the aetiology of otitis media with effusion. Acta Otolaryngol. 2002;122(2):146–52.

63. Hurst DS, Venge P. The impact of atopy on neutrophil activity in middle ear effusion from children and adults with chronic otitis media. Arch Otolaryngol Head Neck Surg. 2002;128(5):561–6.

64. Broides A, et al. Cytology of middle ear fluid during acute otitis media. Pediatr Infect Dis J. 2002;21(1):57–61.

65. Skotnicka B, et al. Lymphocyte subpopulations in middle ear effusions: flow cytometry analysis. Otol Neurotol. 2005;26(4):567–71.

66. Mattila PS, et al. Adenoids provide a microenvironment for the generation of CD4(+), CD45RO(+), L-selectin(−), CXCR4(+), CCR5(+) T lymphocytes, a lymphocyte phenotype found in the middle ear effusion. Int Immunol. 2000;12(9):1235–43.

67. Karjalainen H. Cellular events in relation to bacteria-specific antibodies in middle ear effusion during acute otitis media. Acta Otolaryngol. 1991;111(4):750–5.

68. Ryan AF, et al. Mouse models of induced otitis media. Brain Res. 2006;1091(1):3–8.

69. Jurcisek JA, et al. Anatomy of the nasal cavity in the chinchilla. Cells Tissues Organs. 2003;174(3):136–52.

70. Giebink GS. Otitis media: the chinchilla model. Microb Drug Resist. 1999;5(1):57–72.

71. Bakaletz LO. Chinchilla as a robust, reproducible and polymicrobial model of otitis media and its prevention. Expert Rev Vaccines. 2009;8(8):1063–82.

72. Johnson MD, et al. Murine model of otitis media with effusion: immunohistochemical demonstration of IL-1 alpha antigen expression. Laryngoscope. 1994;104(9):1143–9.

73. Maeda K, et al. Cytokine expression in experimental chronic otitis media with effusion in mice. Laryngoscope. 2004;114(11):1967–72.

74. Stol K, et al. Development of a non-invasive murine infection model for acute otitis media. Microbiology. 2009;155(12):4135–44.

75. Chun YM, et al. Immortalization of normal adult human middle ear epithelial cells using a retrovirus containing the E6/E7 genes of human papillomavirus type 16. Ann Otol Rhinol Laryngol. 2002;111(6):507–17.

76. Sun Y, et al. Activation of p53 transcriptional activity by 1,10-phenanthroline, a metal chelator and redox sensitive compound. Oncogene. 1997;14(4):385–93.

77. Watanabe S, et al. Mutational analysis of human papillomavirus type 16 E7 functions. J Virol. 1990;64(1):207–14.

78. Tsuchiya K, et al. Characterization of a temperature-sensitive mouse middle ear epithelial cell line. Acta Otolaryngol. 2005;125(8):823–9.

79. Herman P, et al. Pathophysiology of middle ear epithelium: a new role for prostaglandin E2. Am J Otolaryngol. 1994;15(4):258–66.

80. Kerschner JE, et al. Mucin gene 19 (MUC19) expression and response to inflammatory cyto-

kines in middle ear epithelium. Glycoconj J. 2009;26(9):1275–84.

81. Choi JY, et al. Ciliary and secretory differentiation of normal human middle ear epithelial cells. Acta Otolaryngol. 2002;122(3):270–5.

82. Clementi CF, Hakansson AP, Murphy TF. Internalization and trafficking of nontypeable *Haemophilus influenzae* in human respiratory epithelial cells and roles of IgA1 proteases for optimal invasion and persistence. Infect Immun. 2014;82(1):433–44.

83. Jalalvand F, et al. *Haemophilus influenzae* protein F mediates binding to laminin and human pulmonary epithelial cells. J Infect Dis. 2013;207(5):803–13.

84. Hallstrom T, et al. *Haemophilus influenzae* protein E binds to the extracellular matrix by concurrently interacting with laminin and vitronectin. J Infect Dis. 2011;204(7):1065–74.

85. Singh B, et al. The unique structure of *Haemophilus influenzae* protein E reveals multiple binding sites for host factors. Infect Immun. 2013;81(3):801–14.

86. Johnson RW, et al. Abrogation of nontypeable *Haemophilus influenzae* protein D function reduces phosphorylcholine decoration, adherence to airway epithelial cells, and fitness in a chinchilla model of otitis media. Vaccine. 2011;29(6):1211–21.

87. Young NM, Foote SJ, Wakarchuk WW. Review of phosphocholine substituents on bacterial pathogen glycans: synthesis, structures and interactions with host proteins. Mol Immunol. 2013;56(4):563–73.

88. Swords WE, et al. Non-typeable Haemophilus influenzae adhere to and invade human bronchial epithelial cells via an interaction of lipooligosaccharide with the PAF receptor. Mol Microbiol. 2000;37(1):13–27.

89. van Schilfgaarde M, et al. Characterization of adherence of nontypeable Haemophilus influenzae to human epithelial cells. Infect Immun. 2000;68(8):4658–65.

90. Lopez-Gomez A, et al. Host cell kinases, alpha5 and beta1 integrins, and Rac1 signalling on the microtubule cytoskeleton are important for non-typable Haemophilus influenzae invasion of respiratory epithelial cells. Microbiology. 2012;158(9):2384–98.

91. Ketterer MR, et al. Infection of primary human bronchial epithelial cells by Haemophilus influenzae: macropinocytosis as a mechanism of airway epithelial cell entry. Infect Immun. 1999;67(8):4161–70.

92. Morey P, et al. Evidence for a non-replicative intracellular stage of nontypable Haemophilus influenzae in epithelial cells. Microbiology. 2011;157(1):234–50.

93. Sharpe SW, Kuehn MJ, Mason KM. Elicitation of epithelial cell-derived immune effectors by outer membrane vesicles of nontypeable Haemophilus influenzae. Infect Immun. 2011;79(11):4361–9.

94. Costerton JW, et al. Bacterial biofilms in nature and disease. Annu Rev Microbiol. 1987;41:435–64.

95. Swords WE. Nontypeable Haemophilus influenzae biofilms: role in chronic airway infections. Front Cell Infect Microbiol. 2012;2:97.

96. MacArthur CJ, et al. Murine middle ear inflammation and ion homeostasis gene expression. Otol Neurotol. 2011;32(3):508–15.

97. Preciado D, et al. NTHi induction of Cxcl2 and middle ear mucosal metaplasia in mice. Laryngoscope. 2013;123(11):E66–71.

98. MacArthur CJ, et al. Otitis media impacts hundreds of mouse middle and inner ear genes. PLoS ONE. 2013;8(10):e75213.

99. Short KR, et al. Influenza-induced inflammation drives pneumococcal otitis media. Infect Immun. 2013;81(3):645–52.

100. MacArthur CJ, et al. Altered expression of middle and inner ear cytokines in mouse otitis media. Laryngoscope. 2011;121(2):365–71.

101. Kariya S, et al. Neutralizing antibody against granulocyte/macrophage colony-stimulating factor inhibits inflammatory response in experimental otitis media. Laryngoscope. 2013;123(6):1514–8.

102. Kariya S, et al. Up-regulation of macrophage migration inhibitory factor induced by endotoxin in experimental otitis media with effusion in mice. Acta Otolaryngol. 2008;128(7):750–5.

103. Eguchi M, et al. Lipopolysaccharide induces proinflammatory cytokines and chemokines in experimental otitis media through the prostaglandin D2 receptor (DP)-dependent pathway. Clin Exp Immunol. 2011;163(2):260–9.

104. Sato K, et al. Middle ear fluid cytokine and inflammatory cell kinetics in the chinchilla otitis media model. Infect Immun. 1999;67(4):1943–6.

105. Hebda PA, et al. Cytokine profiles in a rat model of otitis media with effusion caused by eustachian tube obstruction with and without *Streptococcus pneumoniae* infection. Laryngoscope. 2002;112(9):1657–62.

106. Tong HH, et al. Differential expression of cytokine genes and iNOS induced by nonviable nontypeable *Haemophilus influenzae* or its LOS mutants during acute otitis media in the rat. Int J Pediatr Otorhinolaryngol. 2008;72(8):1183–91.

107. Smirnova MG, et al. Role of the pro-inflammatory cytokines tumor necrosis factor-alpha, interleukin-1 beta, interleukin-6 and interleukin-8 in the pathogenesis of the otitis media with effusion. Eur Cytokine Netw. 2002;13(2):161–72.

108. Himi T, et al. Immunologic characteristics of cytokines in otitis media with effusion. Ann Otol Rhinol Laryngol Suppl. 1992;157:21–5.

109. Tsuchiya K, et al. Interleukin-10 is an essential modulator of mucoid metaplasia in a mouse otitis media model. Ann Otol Rhinol Laryngol. 2008;117(8):630–6.

110. Kurabi A, et al. The inflammasome adaptor ASC contributes to multiple innate immune processes in the resolution of otitis media. Innate Immun, 2014;21(2):203–14.

111. Song JJ, et al. Guggulsterone suppresses LPS induced inflammation of human middle ear epithelial cells (HMEEsC). Int J Pediatr Otorhinolaryngol. 2010;74(12):1384–7.

112. Jono H, et al. Transforming growth factor-beta -Smad signaling pathway cooperates with NF-kappa B to mediate nontypeable *Haemophilus influenzae*-induced MUC2 mucin transcription. J Biol Chem. 2002;277(47):45547–57.

113. Ha U, et al. A novel role for IkappaB kinase (IKK) alpha and IKKbeta in ERK-dependent up-regulation of MUC5AC mucin transcription by *Streptococcus pneumoniae*. J Immunol. 2007;178(3):1736–47.

114. Chen R, et al. Nontypeable *Haemophilus influenzae* lipoprotein P6 induces MUC5AC mucin transcription via TLR2-TAK1-dependent p38 MAPK-AP1 and IKKbeta-IkappaBalpha-NF-kappaB signaling pathways. Biochem Biophys Res Commun. 2004;324(3):1087–94.

115. Tsuboi Y, et al. Induction of mucous cell metaplasia in the middle ear of rats using a three-step method: an improved model for otitis media with mucoid effusion. Acta Otolaryngol. 2002;122(2):153–60.

116. Caye-Thomasen P, Tos M. Histopathologic differences due to bacterial species in acute otitis media. Int J Pediatr Otorhinolaryngol. 2002;63(2):99–110.

117. Caye-Thomasen P, et al. Changes in mucosal goblet cell density in acute otitis media caused by nontypeable *Haemophilus influenzae*. Acta Otolaryngol. 1998;118(2):211–5.

118. Caye-Thomasen P, et al. Changes in goblet cell density in rat middle ear mucosa in acute otitis media. Am J Otol. 1995;16(1):75–82.

119. Hunter SE, et al. Mucin production in the middle ear in response to lipopolysaccharides. Otolaryngol Head Neck Surg. 1999;120(6):884–8.

120. Kerschner JE, et al. Differential response of gel-forming mucins to pathogenic middle ear bacteria. Int J Pediatr Otorhinolaryngol. 2014;78(8): 1368–73.

121. Jono H, et al. Transforming growth factor-beta-Smad signaling pathway negatively regulates nontypeable *Haemophilus influenzae*-induced MUC5AC mucin transcription via mitogen-activated protein kinase (MAPK) phosphatase-1-dependent inhibition of p38 MAPK. J Biol Chem. 2003;278(30):27811–9.

122. Jono H, et al. PKCtheta synergizes with TLR-dependent TRAF6 signaling pathway to upregulate MUC5AC mucin via CARMA1. PLoS ONE. 2012;7(1):e31049.

123. Komatsu K, et al. Glucocorticoids inhibit nontypeable *Haemophilus influenzae*-induced MUC5AC mucin expression via MAPK phosphatase-1-dependent inhibition of p38 MAPK. Biochem Biophys Res Commun. 2008;377(3):763–8.

124. Huang Y, et al. Opposing roles of PAK2 and PAK4 in synergistic induction of MUC5AC mucin by bacterium NTHi and EGF. Biochem Biophys Res Commun. 2007;359(3):691–6.

125. Shen H, et al. Synergistic induction of MUC5AC mucin by nontypeable *Haemophilus influenzae* and *Streptococcus pneumoniae*. Biochem Biophys Res Commun. 2008;365(4):795–800.

126. Lee J, et al. Phosphodiesterase 4B mediates extracellular signal-regulated kinase-dependent up-regulation of mucin MUC5AC protein by Streptococcus pneumoniae by inhibiting cAMP-protein kinase A-dependent MKP-1 phosphatase pathway. J Biol Chem. 2012;287(27):22799–811.

127. Wu X, et al. Human bronchial epithelial cells differentiate to 3D glandular acini on basement membrane matrix. Am J Respir Cell Mol Biol. 2011;44(6):914–21.

128. Catanzaro A, et al. The response to human rIL-1, rIL-2, and rTNF in the middle ear of guinea pigs. Laryngoscope. 1991;101(3):271–5.

129. Watanabe T, et al. Role of interleukin-1beta in a murine model of otitis media with effusion. Ann Otol Rhinol Laryngol. 2001;110(6):574–80.

130. Lee DH, et al. Effect of tumor necrosis factor-alpha on experimental otitis media with effusion. Laryngoscope. 2001;111(4 Pt 1):728–33.

131. Lin J, et al. Induction of mucin gene expression in middle ear of rats by tumor necrosis factor-alpha: potential cause for mucoid otitis media. J Infect Dis. 2000;182(3):882–7.

132. Kawano H, et al. Induction of mucous cell metaplasia by tumor necrosis factor alpha in rat middle ear: the pathological basis for mucin hyperproduction in mucoid otitis media. Ann Otol Rhinol Laryngol. 2002;111(5 Pt 1):415–22.

133. Johnson M, Leonard G, Kreutzer DL. Murine model of interleukin-8-induced otitis media. Laryngoscope. 1997;107(10):1405–8.

134. Kerschner JE, Meyer TK, Burrows A. Chinchilla middle ear epithelial mucin gene expression in response to inflammatory cytokines. Arch Otolaryngol Head Neck Surg. 2004;130(10):1163–7.

135. Choi JY, et al. IL-1beta promotes the ciliogenesis of human middle ear epithelial cells: possible linkage with the expression of mucin gene 8. Acta Otolaryngol. 2005;125(3):260–5.

136. Samuel EA, Burrows A, Kerschner JE. Cytokine regulation of mucin secretion in a human middle ear epithelial model. Cytokine. 2008;41(1):38–43.

137. Nakamura Y, et al. Math1, retinoic acid, and TNF-alpha synergistically promote the differentiation of mucous cells in mouse middle ear epithelial cells in vitro. Pediatr Res. 2013;74(3):259–65.

138. Hirano T, et al. The role of Toll-like receptor 4 in eliciting acquired immune responses against nontypeable *Haemophilus influenzae* following intranasal immunization with outer membrane protein. Int J Pediatr Otorhinolaryngol. 2009;73(12):1657–65.

139. Leichtle A, et al. TLR4-mediated induction of TLR2 signaling is critical in the pathogenesis and resolution of otitis media. Innate Immun. 2009;15(4):205–15.

140. Leichtle A, et al. The role of DNA sensing and innate immune receptor TLR9 in otitis media. Innate Immun. 2012;18(1):3–13.

141. Han F, et al. Role for Toll-like receptor 2 in the immune response to *Streptococcus pneumoniae* infection in mouse otitis media. Infect Immun. 2009;77(7):3100–8.

142. Leichtle A, et al. The toll-Like receptor adaptor TRIF contributes to otitis media pathogenesis and recovery. BMC Immunol. 2009;10:45.

143. Hernandez M, et al. Myeloid differentiation primary response gene 88 is required for the resolution of otitis media. J Infect Dis. 2008;198(12):1862–9.

144. Shuto T, et al. Activation of NF-kappa B by nontypeable *Hemophilus influenzae* is mediated by toll-like receptor 2-TAK1-dependent NIK-IKK alpha/beta-I kappa B alpha and MKK3/6-p38 MAP kinase signaling pathways in epithelial cells. Proc Natl Acad Sci U S A. 2001;98(15):8774–9.

145. Song JJ, et al. Effect of caffeic acid phenethyl ester (CAPE) on H(2)O(2) induced oxidative and inflammatory responses in human middle ear epithelial cells. Int J Pediatr Otorhinolaryngol. 2012;76(5):675–9.

146. Song JJ, et al. Microarray analysis of microRNA expression in LPS induced inflammation of human middle ear epithelial cells (HMEEsCs). Int J Pediatr Otorhinolaryngol. 2011;75(5):648–51.

147. Preciado D, et al. Cigarette smoke activates NFkappaB-mediated Tnf-alpha release from mouse middle ear cells. Laryngoscope. 2010;120(12):2508–15.

148. Martinon F, Tschopp J. Inflammatory caspases and inflammasomes: master switches of inflammation. Cell Death Differ. 2007;14(1):10–22.

149. Ha UH, et al. MKP1 regulates the induction of MUC5AC mucin by *Streptococcus pneumoniae* pneumolysin by inhibiting the PAK4-JNK signaling pathway. J Biol Chem. 2008;283(45):30624–31.

150. Vicente J, et al. Evolution of middle ear changes after permanent eustachian tube blockage. Arch Otolaryngol Head Neck Surg. 2007;133(6):587–92.

151. Zechner G. The condition of the Eustachian tube and its influence on the middle ear. Acta Otolaryngol. 1979;87(3–4):353–61.

152. Kitaoka K, et al. Oxygen consumption by bacteria: a possible cause of negative middle ear pressure in ears with otitis media. Acta Otolaryngol Suppl. 2009;562:63–6.

153. Testa D, et al. Oxidative stress in chronic otitis media with effusion. Acta Otolaryngol. 2012;132(8):834–7.

154. Takoudes TG, J. Haddad J. Evidence of oxygen free radical damage in human otitis media. Otolaryngol Head Neck Surg. 1999;120(5):638–42.

155. Balikci HH, et al. Advanced oxidation protein product level in children with chronic otitis media with effusion. Int J Pediatr Otorhinolaryngol. 2014;78(3):551–3.

156. Huang Q, et al. Hypoxia-inducible factor and vascular endothelial growth factor pathway for the study of hypoxia in a new model of otitis media with effusion. Audiol Neurootol. 2012;17(6):349–56.

157. Cheeseman MT, et al. HIF-VEGF pathways are critical for chronic otitis media in Junbo and Jeff mouse mutants. PLoS Genet. 2011;7(10):e1002336.

158. Bhutta MF, Cheeseman MT, Brown SD. Myringotomy in the Junbo mouse model of chronic otitis media alleviates inflammation and cellular hypoxia. Laryngoscope. 2014;124(9):E377–83.

159. Zhou W, et al. PGI synthase overexpression protects against bleomycin-induced mortality and is associated with increased Nqo 1 expression. Am J Physiol Lung Cell Mol Physiol. 2011;301(4):L615–22.

160. Zhou X, et al. Hypoxia induces mucin expression and secretion in human bronchial epithelial cells. Transl Res. 2012;160(6):419–27.

Diagnosis of Otitis Media

8

Christopher R. Grindle

Introduction

Otitis media with effusion (OME) and acute otitis media (AOM) are exceedingly common diseases, especially in the pediatric population. Most children have experienced at least one episode of AOM by age 3 and by age 6 nearly 40 % have had three infections [1]. Nearly 20 % of all young, school-age children at any given time have middle-ear effusion (MEE)—regardless of source. Otitis media, a catch all term encompassing AOM and OME, is the second most common illness diagnosed in children [2] and the most common reason for children to receive antibiotic therapy [3, 4]. Treatment for OME and AOM is predicated on accurate diagnosis. Increasing effort is being made to be certain of diagnosis of AOM before prescribing antibiotic therapy so as to reduce antibiotic burden and decrease healthcare expenditure. Despite this, there is no gold standard for the diagnosis of AOM or OME. It is a clinical diagnosis with evolving symptoms based on disease state and progression. The purpose of this section is to detail the diagnostic modalities available and demonstrate how they might be used to guide therapeutic intervention.

To properly diagnose otitis media, one must get an adequate view of the middle ear. This is not always easy. In general, the largest speculum possible should be used to examine the ear. This permits the widest possible field of view. The speculum should fit comfortably in and be well seated in the outer, cartilaginous portion of the external auditory canal (EAC). Using a smaller speculum limits the field of view and it is far easier to over-insert the speculum which may result in contact with the bony EAC, which is exquisitely painful. The EAC is often tortuous and gentle posterior traction on the pinna can be used to straighten the EAC and allow for better insertion of the speculum. Additionally, the speculum and/or otoscope should be held in such a way so as to brace it against the patient's head. Thus, with any sudden movements, the speculum and otoscope will move with the patient's head. All of these positioning techniques are aimed at reducing any discomfort associated with the exam. This is especially important in children. It can be difficult to examine infants and young children, proper positioning and technique can help in achieving a successful exam.

The normal tympanic membrane is a three-layered membrane with an outer layer of stratified squamous epithelium, a middle fibrous layer and an inner mucosal layer of cuboidal epithelium contiguous with the middle ear mucosa. It is adult size at birth though its orientation changes dramatically over the first few years of life. At birth it is a nearly horizontal orientation (34° from the horizontal plane) but changes as the

C. R. Grindle (✉)
Division of Otolaryngology—Head and Neck Surgery, University of Connecticut School of Medicine, Connecticut Children's Medical Center, 282 Washington St., Hartford, CT 06106, USA
e-mail: cgrindle@connecticutchildrens.org

D. Preciado (ed.), *Otitis Media: State of the art concepts and treatment*, DOI 10.1007/978-3-319-17888-2_8

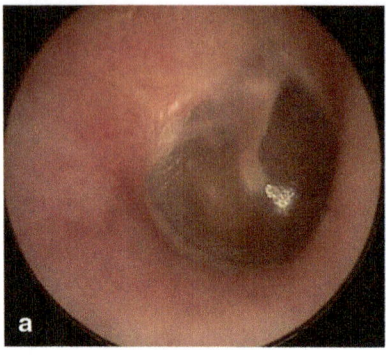 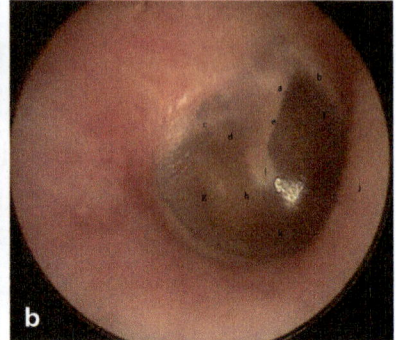

Fig. 8.1 a Otoscopic exam: normal tympanic membrane **b** normal tympanic membrane with landmarks labeled. *a.* lateral process of malleus *b.* tympanic annulus *c.* chorda tympani *d.* incudostapedial joint *e.* handle of malleus *f.* shadow of Eustachian tube *g.* shadow of round window niche *h.* promontory (floor of middle ear) *i.* umbo *j.* bulge of anterior EAC wall *k.* hypotympanic air cells

Table 8.1 Findings on pneumatic otoscopy

Color	Position	Translucency	Mobility
Gray	Normal	Translucent	Normal
Yellow	Bulging	Semiopaque	Increased
Amber	Retracted	Opaque (dull)	Decreased
White			No movement
Red			
Blue			

skull base grows to a more vertical orientation (63° from the horizontal plane) in adults [5]. The normal tympanic membrane is translucent and pearly gray. The malleus (short process and manubrium) can easily be seen. Other landmarks in the middle ear are typically visible through the tympanic membrane (Fig. 8.1a). The most common reasons for the tympanic membrane not to appear normal are OME and AOM. There are many possible findings when examining the tympanic membrane (Table 8.1 and Fig. 8.1b) and good description of the exam findings helps to standardize communication between clinicians.

In contrast to a normal tympanic membrane, the exam findings in otitis media are quite different. OME (Fig. 8.2) will often present with complaints of fullness and possibly decreased hearing. It may also be asymptomatic. Exam findings in serous OME are usually a yellow or amber tympanic membrane with normal or retracted position. Mobility is usually impaired and air bubbles may be seen in the fluid in the

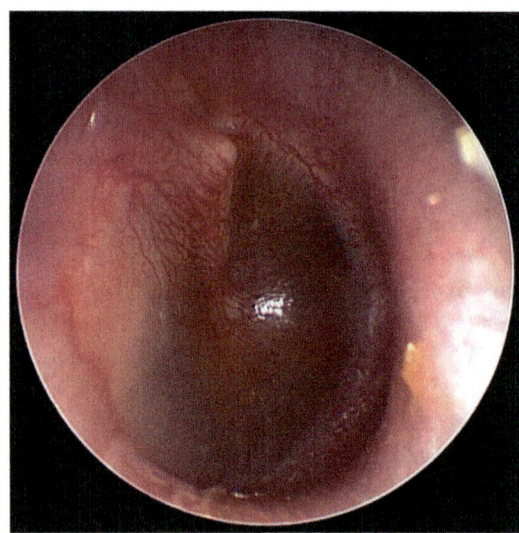

Fig. 8.2 Otoscopic exam: serous otitis media

middle ear space. Mucoid OME has a yellow to white or creamy color with a bulging, normal, or retracted position. Mobility is also usually de-

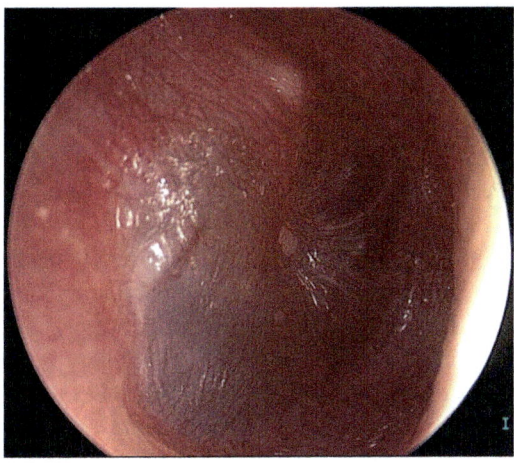

Fig. 8.3 Otoscopic exam: mucoid effusion with bubbles

creased (Fig. 8.3). The findings in OME contrast with the findings in AOM. Here the patient may or may not complain or ear pain. The tympanic membrane will be red with prominent vessels. There will be effusion in the middle ear space, often purulent in appearance, and the tympanic membrane will appear in a normal or bulging position. Mobility will also likely be decreased (Fig. 8.4).

Of paramount importance is making the correct diagnosis for a patient with otitis media as the diagnosis will determine the treatment. The 2013 Clinical practice guideline: Diagnosis and

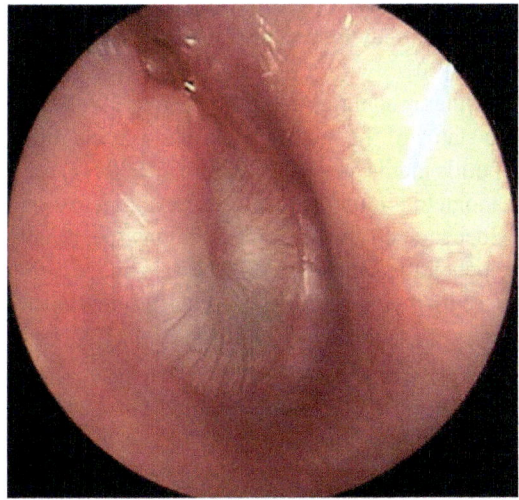

Fig. 8.4 Otoscopic exam: AOM

Management of AOM from the American Academy of Pediatrics (AAP) [6] built upon and further clarified diagnostic criteria set forth in the 2004 AAP guidelines [7]. The 2004 guidelines used a three part definition of AOM with (1) acute onset of symptoms, (2) presence of MEE, and (3) signs of middle ear inflammation. Criticisms of these criteria were that they lacked precision to exclude OME and permitted the diagnosis of AOM in cases of acute onset of symptoms with otlagia and MEE but without other signs of inflammation on otoscopy. Additionally, the 2004 guidelines included a category for "uncertain diagnosis" which may have permitted diagnosis of AOM without clear visualization of the tympanic membrane. The 2013 guidelines qualify these criteria and states that the diagnosis of AOM:

1. Should be made in children who present with moderate to severe bulging of the tympanic membrane (TM) or new onset otorrhea not due to acute otitis externa
2. Should be made in children who present with mild bulging of the TM *and* recent onset (less than 48 h) of ear pain (holding, tugging, and rubbing of the ear in a nonverbal child) or intense erythema of the TM
3. Should *not* be made in children who do not have MEE (based on pneumatic otoscopy and/or tympanometry)

Critically, the new guidelines place great importance on the otoscopic exam of the patient to make the correct diagnosis. A study by Karma et al. [8] looked at over 2900 children over the course of 2 years at two separate sites—totaling over 11,000 visits. Physical exam findings, the color, position, and the mobility of the TM were recorded. AOM was diagnosied if the child had MEE and fever, earache, irritability, ear rubbing or tugging simultaneous other upper respiratory symptoms, vomiting, or diarrhea. Tympanocentesis was performed but no culture was obtained. Of the acute visits in the study, MEE was found in 84.9 and 81.8% at the two sites. Of the exam findings, a cloudy, bulging TM with impaired mobility was the best predictor of AOM. Impaired mobility had the highest sensitivity (95%) and specificity

(85%). Individually, cloudiness was 74% sensitive and 93% specific. Bulging TM was only 51% sensitive, but 97% specific. Several other studies support the value of the bulging TM on physical exam [9, 10] moderate to severe bulging of the TM is the most important characteristic in the diagnosis of AOM [6].

In looking at the presenting symptoms of AOM, ear pain had the highest combined positive likelihood ratio (3.0–7.3) in a 2003 review by Rothman et al. [11]. In three studies cited, Niemela et al. reported 54% sensitivity and 82% specificity of ear pain [12]. Heikkinen reported 60% sensitivity and 92% specificity [13] and Ingvarrson reported 100% sensitivity, though did not report specificity [14].

Despite its usefulness as a symptom to be used in the diagnosis of AOM, ear pain is only present in 50–60% of children with AOM [11]. Other signs, restless, ear rubbing, fever, non-specific respiratory complaints, diarrhea do not appear to be helpful in the diagnosis of AOM.

Takata et al. reviewed the accuracy of eight methods of diagnosing OME [15]. Pneumatic otoscopy was found to have the best performance with a sensitivity of 94% (95% CI 92–96%) and a specificity of 80% (95% CI 75–86%). Pneumatic otoscopy was compared to acoustic reflectometer, portable tympanometry and several variations of professional tympanometry. All included studies used myringotomy as internal diagnostic comparison. Only one of the included studies on pneumatic otoscopy was performed by validated otoscopists [16]. Additionally, the author notes that audiometry, binocular microscopy and nonpneumatic otoscopy could not be included in the analysis because of inadequate evidence. In a small study, Rogers et al. looked at 201 ears in 102 patients and found that binocular by a staff pediatric otolaryngologist was the most sensitive in diagnosing OME with 88.0% sensitivity (95% CI 81.4–94.7) and 89% specificity (95% CI 83.1–94.9). Resident binocular microscopy was the next most sensitive, followed by staff pneumatic otoscopy and resident pneumatic otoscopy. Thus, as would be expected, there is improved performance garnered from additional years of training and experience. Interestingly, however, even the resident exam was more specific that the tympanometer 78.4% (95% CI 70.4–86.4) to 47.7% (95% CI 38.3–57.1).

Tympanometry

Tympanograms are widely used as an adjunct to the pneumatic otoscope in the clinical evaluation of children with otitis media. Most primary care clinics today use a low-frequency probe tones (220–226 Hz) [17] and classify results as Jerger A, B, or C [18]. Type A represents normal compliance of the tympanic membrane, type B no compliance and type C negative pressure in the middle ear space. Tympanometry with low-frequency probe is reliable for infants greater than 4 months and has good interobserver agreement of the curve patterns in routine clinical practice [19]. Despite the relatively low specificity, 47.7% in the Rogers study and 74.5% in the Takata study for predicting MEE with a type B tympanogram can guide the clinician in clinical decision-making. If the definition of abnormal results on tympanogram are expanded to include both type B as well as type C2 (tympanic peak pressures between −200 and −400 daPa) the sensitivity and specificity, according to data from Takata, improve to 93.8% (95% CI 91.1–96.4) and 61.8% (95% CI 41.5–82.1), respectively. Although not as precise as pneumatic otoscopy, this definition of abnormal result may be the most useful for ruling out OME [20].

Other modalities that have been used to assess the status of the middle ear and aid in diagnosis of otitis media are high frequenct (1000 Hz) tympanometry, multifrequency tympanometry, and wideband acoustic transfer functions specifically wideband reflectance (WBR). Data suggest that these methods are useful in specific situations to determine the presence or absence of MEE, especially 1000 Hz tympanometry and WBR as applied to screening in infants. Continued research is needed to define their exact role as diagnostic tools [20]. Acoustic reflectometry (AR) is another tool that can be used in the diagnosis of MEE. Modern acoustic reflectometers analyze the frequency spectrum of reflected sound. They have been shown to be nearly equivalent to pneumatic otoscopy and tympanometry in terms of sensitivity and specificity [21]. AR offers a potential advantage over tympanometry and pneumatic otoscopy in that it does not require an airtight seal. AR, however, is not widely available for clinical use at this time.

Hearing Testing

Audiometry may be used in the assessment of patients with otitis media. It is recommended when MEE has been present for 3 months or greater or when there is concern for speech delay, learning problems or when a significant hearing loss is suspected. Audiometric results with otitis can range from normal to moderate hearing loss (0–55 dB). The average hearing loss is 25 dB hearing level (HL) and approximately 20% of ears exceed 35 dB HL [19]. The hearing loss is conductive in nature and secondary to the effusion in the middle ear space or the retraction of the TM. It causes an overall stiffening of the middle ear transduction mechanism (TM and ossicles) that generally affect lower frequencies before higher frequencies [22].

Conventional audiometry can be performed for children greater than 4 years of age. Screening conventional audiometry can be performed in the primary care setting. For younger children and for those for whom conventional audiometry is not appropriate, comprehensive audiologic assessment should be obtained. This includes air conduction and bone conduction thresholds for pure tones, speech detection and speech reception thresholds. For children aged 6–24 months, visual reinforced audiometry may be used. Play audiometry is typically used for children 24–48 months [23]. Assessment of individual ear thresholds using either headphones or in canal inserts is typically possible with children older than 24 months. If this is not possible, then assessment is done under soundfield conditions and the responses can only comment on the better hearing ear.

Auditory brainstem response (ABR) testing and otoacoustic emission (OAE) testing are not tests of hearing but rather assessments of the integrity of the auditory pathway. They are objective measures used in situations wherein behavioral testing is not possible (e.g., newborn screening), but they should not be used as a substitute for behavioral audiometry [23].

Impact of Correct Diagnosis

The correct diagnosis of otitis media drives all further management of the patient. Decisions regarding treatment and follow-up, discussed elsewhere in this book, are all based upon diagnosis. Since the introduction of the 2004 AAP guidelines [7] several studies have examined their effect on diagnosis and treatment. AOM is the most common diagnosis for which antibiotics were prescribed for children less than 6 years of age [24]. However, in the initial years after the publication of the 2004 guidelines, there was a drop in the proportion of visits that resulted in antibiotic from 66.0% in 2005 to 51.9% in 2007. This trend was followed by an increase in proportion over the subsequent years to pre guideline levels. There was a second decrease in antibiotic prescriptions beginning in 2010 with 2011 levels at 57.6%. Additionally, 54% of the prescriptions were for amoxicillin—keeping with the guideline recommendations [25]. Vaz et al. [24] also reported a decrease in the antibiotic prescriptions for AOM comparing rates in 2000–2001 and 2009–2010. They note that the decreases were driven by decreases in the frequency of diagnosis of AOM. There were only modest changes in the management once AOM was diagnosed. This finding may be due to the increased focus on correct diagnosis in the 2004 guideline. The 2013 AAP guidelines [6] continue to refine the diagnosis of AOM with the addition of strict otoscopic criteria and clarification of areas of uncertainty. This may result in even further reduction in the number of AOM diagnoses and prescribed antibiotics.

Conclusion

The diagnosis of otitis media can be difficult for even the most experienced of clinicians. It is a disease that primarily affects younger children who can be difficult to examine at best. Additionally, there is no gold standard for diagnosis of otitis media. Recent studies and guidelines continue to refine the diagnostic criteria, with significant emphasis on physical exam findings, so as to help the clinician make an accurate diagnosis which informs all other decisions of therapy and management.

References

1. Casselbrant ML, Mandel EM. Epidemiology. In: Rosenfeld RM, Bluestone CD, editors. Evidence-Based otitis media. 2. ed. Hamilton: BC Decker; 2003. p. 147–62.
2. Centers for Disease Control and Prevention. Table 2: top 5 diagnoses at visits to office-based physicians and hospital outpatient departments by patient age and sex: United States 2008. In: National Ambulatory Health Care Survey 2008. Atlanta: Centers for Disease Control and Prevention; 2008.
3. Grijalva CG, Nuorti JP, Griffin MR. Antibiotic prescription rates for acute respiratory tract infections in US ambulatory settings. JAMA. 2009;302(7):758–66.
4. McCaig LF, Besser RE, Hughes JM. Trends in antimicrobial prescribing rates for children and adolescents. JAMA. 2002;287(23):3096–102.
5. Isaacson G. Endoscopic anatomy of the pediatric middle ear. Otolaryngol Head Neck Surg. 2014;150(1):6–15.
6. Lieberthal AS, Carroll AE, Chonmaitree T, et al. The diagnosis and management of acute otitis media. Pediatrics. 2013;131(3):e964–99.
7. American Academy of Pediatrics Sub-committee on Management of Acute Otitis Media. Diagnosis and management of acute otitis media. Pediatrics. 2004;113(5):1451–65.
8. Karma PH, Penttilä MA, Sipilä MM, Kataja MJ. Otoscopic diagnosis of middle eareffusion in acute and non-acute otitismedia. I. The value of different otoscopic findings. Int J Pediatr Otorhinolaryngol. 1989;17(1):37–49.
9. McCormick DP, Lim-Melia E, Saeed K, Baldwin CD, Chonmaitree T. Otitis media: can clinical findings predict bacterial or viral etiology? Pediatr Infect Dis J. 2000;19(3):256–8.
10. Schwartz RH, Stool SE, Rodriguez WJ, Grundfast KM. Acute otitis media: toward a more precise definition. Clin Pediatr (Phila). 1981;20(9):549–54.
11. Rothman R, Owens T, Simel DL. Does this child have acute otitis media? JAMA. 2003;290(12):1633–40.
12. Niemela M, Uhari M, Jounio-Ervasti K, Luotonen J, Alho OP, Vierimaa E. Lack of specific symptomatology in children with acute otitis media. Pediatr Infect Dis J. 1994;13(9):765–8.
13. Heikkinen T, Ruuskanen O. Signs and symptoms predicting acute otitis media. Arch Pediatr Adolesc Med. 1995;149(1):26–9.
14. Ingvarsson L. Acute otalgia in children—findings and diagnosis. Acta Paediatr Scand. 1982;71(5):705–10.
15. Takata GS, Chan LS, Morphew T, Mangione-Smith R, Morton SC, Shekelle P. Evidence assessment of the accuracy of methods of diagnosing middle ear effusion in children with otitis media with effusion. Pediatrics. 2003 Dec;112(6 Pt 1):1379–87.
16. Paradise JL, Smith CG, Bluestone CD. Tympanometric detection of middle ear effusion in infants and young children. Pediatrics. 1976;58:198–210.
17. Johnson KC. Audiologic assessment of children with suspected hearing loss. Otolaryngol Clin N Am. 2002;35(4):711–32.
18. Jerger JF. Clinical experience with impedence audiometry. Arch Otolaryngol. 1970;92:311–24.
19. Rosenfeld RM, Culpepper L, Doyle KJ, Grundfast KM, Hoberman A, Kenna MA, et al. Clinical practice guideline: otitis media with effusion. Otolaryngol Head Neck Surg. 2004;130(Suppl. 5):S95–118.
20. Sanford CA, Schooling T, Frymark T. Determining the presence or absence of middle ear disorders: an evidence-based systematic review on the diagnostic accuracy of selected assessment instruments. Am J Audiol. 2012;21:251–68.
21. Teppo H, Revonta M. Comparison of old, professional and consumer model acoustic reflectometers in the detection of middle-ear fluid in children with recurrent acute otitis media or glue ear. Int J Pediatr Otorhinolaryngol. 2007;71:1855–72.
22. Stach BA. Audiologic evaluation of otologic/neurotologic disease. In: Gulya AJ, Minor LB, Poe DS, editors. Glasscock, Shambaugh, Surgery of the ear. 6. ed. Connecticut:People's Medical Publishing House; 2010. p. 189–221.
23. Cunningham M. AAP clinical report hearing assessment in infant and children. Pediatrics. 2003;111:436–40.
24. Vaz LE, Kleinman KP, Raebel MA, Nordin JD, Lakoma MD, Dutta-Linn MM, Finkelstein JA. Recent trends in outpatient antibiotic use in children. Pediatrics. 2014;133(3):375–85. doi:10.1542/peds.2013-2903. (Epub 2014 Feb 2).
25. McGrath LJ, Becker-Dreps S, Pate V, Brookhart MA. Trends in antibiotic treatment of acute otitis media and treatment failure in children, 2000–2011. PLoS ONE. 2013;8(12):e81210. doi:10.1371/journal.pone.0081210.

Part III
Treatments

Treatment: Impact of Vaccination and Progress in Vaccine Development

Laura A. Novotny and Lauren O. Bakaletz

List of Abbreviations

AOM	Acute otitis media
EPS	Extracellular polymeric substance
NTHI	Nontypeable *Haemophilus influenzae*
OM	Otitis media
PD	Protein D
RSV	Respiratory syncytial virus
URI	Upper respiratory tract infection

Current Vaccination Recommendations

The vaccination schedule for pediatric patients is designed to deliver vaccines to this highly vulnerable population at intervals intended to optimally protect them against infectious diseases. Set by the Centers for Disease Control and Prevention and based on recommendations from the Advisory Committee on Immunization Practices, these practices are reviewed and revised annually to ensure that the guidelines concur with the current recommendations for licensed vaccines and to incorporate newly released formulations.

L. O. Bakaletz (✉)
Department of Pediatrics, The Research Institute at Nationwide Children's Hospital, Ohio State University College of Medicine, 700 Children's Drive, W591, Columbus, OH 43205, USA
e-mail: lauren.bakaletz@nationwidechildrens.org

L. A. Novotny
Department of Pediatrics, The Research Institute at Nationwide Children's Hospital, Center for Microbial Pathogensis, Columbus, OH, USA

At present, although a vaccine designed specifically for the prevention of otitis media (OM) does not exist, several vaccine formulations are currently licensed that contain components to target two of the predominant bacterial causative agents of OM, *Streptococcus pneumoniae* and nontypeable *Haemophilus influenzae* (NTHI). Although primarily indicated for the prevention of invasive disease caused by *S. pneumoniae*, these formulations, by extension, are shown to reduce the number of episodes of OM in the pediatric population [1].

The first of these interventions was made available in 2000, when a 7-valent pneumococcal conjugate vaccine (PCV7; Prevnar™/Prevenar™) manufactured by Wyeth Vaccines was licensed for use by the Food and Drug Administration. Targeting the seven most prevalent strains of *S. pneumoniae* in North America [2], PCV7 incorporated capsular polysaccharides from pneumococcal serotypes 4, 6B, 9V, 14, 18C, 19F, and 7F, each conjugated to CRM_{197}, a nontoxic variant of diphtheria toxin from *Corynebacterium diphtheriae*. This vaccine was approved for use in children 2–24 months of age, and administered as a primary series of three doses delivered intramuscularly at 2, 4, and 6 months of age, and boosted at 12–15 months [3].

In an effort to provide broader and more global pneumococcal serotype coverage, a second generation 13-valent pneumococcal conjugate vaccine (PCV13) from Pfizer received licensing approval in 2010 [2]. In addition to the *S. pneumoniae* serotypes targeted with the heptavalent formulation, PCV13 incorporated additional capsular polysaccharides to provide coverage for pneumococcal serotypes 1, 3, 5, 6A, 7F, and 19A, each conjugated to CRM_{197}. For children that had not yet received either pneumococcal conjugate vaccine, PCV13 is recommended to be administered at 2, 4, and 6 months of age, and boosted at 12–15 months. Healthy children between 14 and 59 months of age who completed the PCV7 series are advised to receive a single dose PCV13, while it is recommended that children with underlying medical conditions are administered two doses prior to 71 months of age [4].

Due to the emergence of invasive pneumococcal strains of increasing prevalence in developing countries not included in the prior pneumococcal conjugate vaccine formulations and to further expand serotype coverage, a decavalent conjugate vaccine (PHiD-CV/Synflorix™) manufactured by GlaxoSmithKline was approved for use in Canada and Australia in 2008 and in the European Union in 2009 [5]. PHiD-CV incorporates capsular polysaccharides from pneumococcal serotypes 1, 4, 5, 6B, 7F, 9V, 14, 18C, 19F, and 23F. While tetanus toxoid and diphtheria toxoid serve as carrier molecules for two of the included pneumococcal serotypes (18C and 19F, respectively), to address concerns of interference with coadministered conjugate vaccines, protein D from NTHI is conjugated to pneumococcal polysaccharides from serotypes 1, 5, 6B, 7F, 9V, 14, and 23F. PHiD-CV is currently indicated for invasive pneumococcal disease and pneumonia in infants, and as an additional benefit, inclusion of Protein D is shown to provide protection against OM due to NTHI [6]. It is recommended that infants are administered PHiD-CV at 2, 4, and 6 months of age, and boosted at 12–15 months, or alternatively, 2, 4, and 11–12 months of age.

Impact on Prevalence and Complications Associated with Use of Pneumococcal Conjugate Vaccines

For OM due to *S. pneumoniae*, the release of PCV7 in 2000 resulted in a welcome 69–91 % decrease in invasive pneumococcal disease.

However, despite also being associated with both a 56–57 % decrease in acute OM (AOM) associated with the pneumococcal serotypes included in the vaccine [7–9], and a notable reduction in tympanostomy tube insertion [10], PCV7 yielded an only modest overall decrease in AOM (~6–7 %) [11].

Importantly, near universal PCV7 adoption in the USA, along with the later release of a PCV13, as well as PHiD-CV [5, 12–14] resulted in a significant change in the microbiology of AOM [7, 11, 15–18]. There has been an increase in AOM due to non-vaccine serotypes of Spn (i.e., a phenomenon referred to as "serotype replacement") [19–22] and a considerable increase in the proportion of cases of OM caused by NTHI and *Moraxella catarrhalis*. Globally, NTHI is now as important a causative agent of AOM as *S. pneumoniae* [1, 23]. Moreover, in a recent survey of bacteria cultured from the middle ears of children, NTHI was the most frequently isolated bacterium from those who failed treatment [24]. There is clearly still a great need for post-licensure monitoring with regard to current vaccines for *S. pneumoniae*-induced OM, but also an obligation to consider non-capsular vaccine antigens [25].

Vaccines for NTHI, Where Are We?

In 2006, the results of the Pneumococcal Otitis Efficacy Trial (POET) study [6] demonstrated for the first time that one could immunize parenterally against OM due to NTHI. As mentioned earlier, in this first study, NTHI outer membrane protein D (PD) was conjugated to capsular polysaccharide of 11 serotypes of Spn (called "Pnc-PD"). Efficacy of ~57 % versus AOM due to Spn was obtained, which was very similar to that shown by the already licensed PCV7. However, the efficacy against *all* AOM was 34 %, far greater than the 6–7 % reported for PCV7. Moreover, POET data revealed that Pnc-PD also demonstrated 35.3 % efficacy versus AOM due to NTHI, and a 41.4 % reduction in nasopharyngeal (NP) carriage of NTHI [6], a result attributed to the inclusion of an NTHI-specific antigen in Pnc-PD [26]. This study generated significant enthusiasm in the research community that had been endeavoring to determine if one could indeed immunize against NTHI-induced OM, however, the demonstration of efficacy against approximately one third of NTHI-induced OM, lead to the broadly held belief that additional NTHI antigens are needed to improve coverage for NTHI-induced OM [27]. This is due to both the relatively limited efficacy shown and the fact that there is vast heterogeneity amongst NTHI isolates, thus the exclusive use of any single antigen in a vaccine to prevent NTHI-induced OM is unlikely to be sufficient. Since the POET study, and following release of a 10-valent version of Pnc-PD (PHiD-CV) [5], an additional study on NP colonization after immunization in the second year of life demonstrated no effect on colonization by NTHI or any other pathogen [13]. Moreover, as a follow-up to the licensure of PHiD-CV, Smith-Vaughan et al. assessed multiple carriage and disease isolates of NTHI and reported the absence of the gene that encodes PD in ~19% [28]. The inability of ~19% of NTHI isolates to express PD (the antigen targeted by PHiD-CV) helps to explain the limited ~35% efficacy against AOM due to NTHI in the POET study, and solidifies the need for vaccines directed against NTHI-induced OM to include multiple antigens.

As to which NTHI antigens to consider, this has been the subject of much discussion and research by many laboratories. Those for which significant progress had been made were recently summarized in a report of the Vaccine Panel convened immediately following the 2011 *10th International Symposium on Recent Advances in Otitis Media* [29]. Included in this revised "short list" are now only seven antigens: OMP P6, protein D, detoxified lipooligosaccharide, HMW1/HMW2, Hia, OMP P5-derived peptides, and PilA. While work continues on the development of these and other vaccine candidates for the prevention of NTHI-induced OM, progression forward to human clinical trials is indeed what is needed for those that have already been extensively tested both *in vitro* and in animal models.

Future Directions in Vaccination Efforts

Beyond those advances already mentioned above, future directions in vaccination efforts for OM include: (1) the targeting of viral coinfections, (2) development of pneumococcal proteins as vaccine candidates in addition to capsular polysaccharides, (3) ongoing efforts at antigen discovery for the third predominant bacterial pathogen of OM—*M. catarrhalis*, (4) investigation of the bacterial biofilms in an attempt to identify biofilm-focused determinants for the development of not only traditional preventative vaccine candidates but also those that might resolve existing OM, and (5) development of noninvasive methods to immunize against OM, thus potentially increasing both compliance and access to these vaccines. A brief summary of each is provided below.

Targeting of Viral Coinfections

Viral upper respiratory tract infections (URI), either preceding or concurrent, is the most common predisposing factor for bacterial OM and as such protection against viral URI has been a long-held strategy for protection against OM. To date, evidence in support of this assertion is available for vaccines against influenza A virus only [30], however multiple respiratory tract viruses are associated with the development of bacterial OM. In addition to influenza A virus, the most common are respiratory syncytial virus (RSV), human rhinovirus, and adenovirus. There are active efforts to develop vaccines against RSV as well as other viral co-pathogens of OM, however antigenic diversity amongst strains and the lack of appropriate animal models are considered major barriers to progress in this regard. In addition to predisposing to bacterial invasion of the middle ear via a variety of mechanisms, prolonged AOM and antibiotic treatment failure are associated with concurrent viral infection. Thus, the targeting of viral coinfections for vaccine development efforts to prevent OM remains an active and important area of investigation.

Development of Pneumococcal Proteins as Vaccine Candidates

Despite the success of conjugated polysaccharide vaccines which have greatly reduced the global burden of pneumococcal diseases, including pneumococcal OM, the observations of increasing disease due to replacement serotypes and differences in distribution of serotypes responsible for disease worldwide [31] strongly suggest that any vaccine that provides coverage for a limited number of serotypes will not provide the needed long-term solution for protection against pneumococcal OM. As such, there is an effort to identify and test broadly conserved pneumococcal protein antigens that could, in theory, provide serotype-independent protection. Moreover, it is likely that these vaccines would not induce serotype replacement, and further, believed to be much less costly to produce than the current conjugated capsular polysaccharide vaccines. Several candidates are currently being investigated in this regard, including: pneumococcal surface protein A (PspA), histidine triad family (Pht), pneumococcal surface adhesin A (PsaA), pneumococcal type 1 and type 2 pilus subunits, pneumolysin, pneumococcal serine-rich repeat protein (PsrP), pneumococcal choline binding protein (PcpA), heat shock protein caseinolytic protease (Clp), sortase A (SrtA), polyamine transport operon (potD), pneumococcal protective protein (PppA), a protein analogous to the cell wall separation protein of group B streptococcus (PcsB), and a serine/threonine protein kinase (StkP), among others. These candidates cannot be discussed fully here, however several excellent reviews are available for interested readers [29, 32]. Recently, Berglund et al. [25] reported the results of a phase I clinical trial in adults, in which a protein-based NTHI and pneumococcal vaccine that contained pneumococcal histidine triad D (PhtD), detoxified pneumolysin (dPly), and NTHI protein D was tested, thereby demonstrating significant forward momentum in

continued vaccine development wherein two predominant pathogens of OM, as well as multiple other diseases of the airway are targeted.

Antigen Discovery for *M. catarrhalis*

M. catarrhalis has always been considered the third ranking bacterial agent of OM, after *S. pneumoniae* and NTHI, however the recent shift in the microbiology of OM resulting from the broad use of pneumococcal conjugate vaccines has now resulted in an increase in the relative role of both NTHI and *M. catarrhalis* in OM. As a result, there has been much progress recently in attempts to identify potential vaccine antigens that target *M. catarrhalis*. A genome mining approach has been particularly fruitful in this regard and as such, several new and promising candidates have emerged. Currently, the following potential antigens are under development: MID/Hag; MchA1 & MchA2; MhaB1 & MhaB2; McmA; OppA, UspA2, Msp75; McaP; OMP E; OMP CD; M35; OMP G1a & OMP G1b; OlpA; Msp 22, Type IV pili; and lipooligosaccharide [29, 33]. Although limitations in availability of relevant animal models in which to test *M. catarrhalis*-derived vaccine candidates has slowed progress in the past, use of the murine pulmonary clearance model [34] and a newly developed chinchilla polymicrobial model wherein RSV predisposes to invasion of the middle ear by both NTHI and *M. catarrhalis* [35] are being used to move these candidates forward.

Identification of Biofilm-focused Determinants

By definition, a biofilm is a highly organized, multicellular community encased in an extracellular polymeric matrix or substance (often referred to as the EPS) that is affixed to a surface. Biofilms are the preferred state of all bacterial lifestyles in nature. Bacteria populations within a biofilm, as opposed to their planktonic or free-living counterparts, have a reduced growth rate (due to a nutrient limited environment), and a distinct transcriptome [36, 37]. They also exchange genetic material at an increased frequency. Bacteria in a biofilm have *substantially increased* resistance not only to effectors of innate and acquired immunity but also to the action of antibiotics [38–40]. Moreover, the EPS presents a formidable physical barrier to cellular effectors of immunity and is highly recalcitrant to removal [41]. Diseases wherein there is a biofilm component as part of the disease course, such as OM, thus require novel methods for diagnosis, treatment, and prevention. The biofilm paradigm was originally put forth because OM is a spectrum of diseases that are very difficult to treat with antibiotics and are often chronic and recurrent in nature. Moreover, effusions recovered from middle ears are often bacteriologically sterile. However, although bacteria cannot be cultured from these effusions, they are nonetheless typically PCR-positive for bacterial DNA [42]. Moreover, Rayner et al. [42] demonstrated that, in addition to bacterial DNA, there was also bacterial *messenger* RNA present in middle ear fluids. The presence of this short-lived message suggested the existence of metabolically active bacteria within those fluids, despite an inability to culture them. To date, all three major otopathogens—*S. pneumoniae*, NTHI, and *M. catarrhalis*—have been shown to form biofilms both *in vitro* and *in vivo* [43–47]. Direct detection of bacterial biofilms in association with mucosa samples recovered from the middle ears of children with chronic and recurrent OM has been shown [48]. Current data support the role of biofilms in recurrent and chronic OM, however, it would be counterintuitive to not consider the possibility that biofilms also contribute to AOM as bacteria require only minutes to begin building a biofilm in a favorable environment.

Due to the unique and highly resistant of bacteria resident within a biofilm, many in the research community are attempting to better characterize these biofilms, as well as understand the molecular mechanisms and microenvironmental cues that trigger their development/dispersal so that novel methods to target them for either disruption or immune intervention can be developed [49–55].

Development of Noninvasive Immunization Routes

Another significant challenge to development of vaccines for OM is the already extremely crowded recommended pediatric immunization schedule [56]. An infant in developed countries receives no less than 8–11 injections in the first year of life [57], with typically 4–5 injections per visit. Worldwide, there are concerns about reduced compliance due to parental anxiety over the "pin-cushion" status of their newborns, as well as scientific concerns about the potential for immune interference, particularly when multiple vaccines are formulated with common carriers. This state of pediatric immunization practice is leading to two significant developments in the pediatric vaccine industry. The first is an emphasis on the development of combination vaccines, to reduce the total number of injections received [58, 59]. However, there is also tremendous interest and emphasis being put on the development of alternative delivery strategies, and particularly the use of noninvasive or "needle-free" routes of immunization [60–63]. There are multiple advantages to noninvasive routes of immunization in general, including the fact that they eliminate the pain, anxiety, and aversion associated with injection, thus yielding better compliance; they eliminate the use of needles and thereby both increase safety and eradicate the need to dispose of medical "sharps" waste; they are typically much cheaper to produce and less likely to require a "cold chain" due to their greater stability and longer shelf life; and the fact that for many of these delivery regimes, trained medical personnel are not required. With regard to mucosal diseases such as OM, the primary and perhaps critical advantage of noninvasive vaccination routes is that unlike parenteral immunization, these approaches induce the formation of both mucosal and systemic immunity, thereby facilitating the availability of a robust, protective response at the exact site of bacterial colonization/infection, and thus precisely where it is needed the most.

Mucosal immunization has become one area of great developing interest in the OM community [64, 65]. Further, recent publications report efficacy against experimental OM due to NTHI after immunizing transcutaneously (by rubbing the vaccine candidate onto the skin of the chinchilla ear) [66, 67]. Not only was this approach protective against the development of experimental OM but was also efficacious as a therapeutic vaccine, mediating significantly more rapid resolution of existing disease. Collectively, these efforts will not only help de-crowd the pediatric immunization schedule but they also have the potential for even greater efficacy than can be achieved by traditional immunization routes. Fostering a local immune response may also prove to provide greater protection to those targeted groups wherein there are genetic and/or anatomical risk factors for proneness to OM (i.e., Native Americans, Alaskan Natives, Aboriginal peoples, those with Down's syndrome, or with cleft lip/palate, among others) [68–70].

Does It Matter?

The answer to this, in our opinion, is an unequivocal "yes." OM remains *the most common bacterial disease of childhood*, with substantial public health implications [71–75]. OM is the primary cause for emergency room visits [72] and is the most frequently diagnosed illness in children under 15 years of age, although peak incidence of disease is between 9 and 15 months [76]. It is estimated that 709 million cases of AOM and 65–330 million episodes of chronic secretory OM occur each year worldwide, with the greatest burden of disease experienced by children under age 4 [77, 78]. While mortality due to OM is not common in developed countries, it is nonetheless still responsible for ~28,000 deaths per year in the developing world [79], and the attendant morbidity of OM is significant for *all* children. OM is also *the most common cause of hearing loss in childhood*, an outcome associated with developmental delays in behavior, language, and education for this very young population [80–84]. Where available, antibiotic use has historically been heavily relied upon for medical management of OM [17, 74, 85], in fact, worldwide, treatment of AOM is among the greatest drivers of antibiotic use in children [29]. Moreover,

chronic OM is typically very difficult to resolve, often requiring prolonged antibiotic treatment, which is of great concern due to the resulting sobering emergence of multiple antibiotic-resistant bacteria in all three genera of bacteria that predominate in OM [86, 87]. This alarming increase in resistance to antimicrobials is not surprising when one considers that antibiotic use in children is more than three times that in any other age group, and in fact, 40 % of all outpatient antibiotic use in children is for treatment of OM [72, 88].

Surgical management of chronic OM involves the insertion of tympanostomy tubes while a child is under general anesthesia and is *the most common ambulatory surgery procedure for children in the USA*. While highly effective in terms of relieving painful symptoms by draining the middle ear of accumulated fluids, tube insertion has met with criticism due to its invasive nature and the incumbent risks of putting a child under general anesthesia [74, 89–92]. The socioeconomic impact of OM is great. Total direct and indirect costs of AOM in non-vaccinated preschool children is $3.8 billion [93], whereas that for management of OM overall, exceeds $5 billion annually in the USA alone [74, 94–96]. Although serious complications of OM such as brain abscess, mastoiditis, meningitis, epidural abscess, and sinus thrombosis are rare, other sequelae of OM such as TM perforation and atelectasis of the TM are quite common [97]. Inner ear sequelae can cause hearing loss (in addition to the conductance type of hearing loss associated with the presence of fluid, pus and/or biofilms within the middle ear that impede action of the ossicles) as well as speech and language problems. Clearly, there is a tremendous need to develop more effective and accepted approaches to the management and preferably, the *prevention* of OM.

References

1. Haggard M. Otitis media: prospects for prevention. Vaccine. 2008;26(Suppl 7):G20-4. PMID: 19094934.
2. Grijalva CG, Pelton SI. A second-generation pneumococcal conjugate vaccine for prevention of pneumococcal diseases in children. Curr Opin Pediatr. 2011;23(1):98–104. PMID: 21191300.

3. Centers for Disease Control and Prevention. Advisory Committee on Immunization Practices. Updated recommendation from the Advisory Committee on Immunization Practices (ACIP) for use of 7-valent pneumococcal conjugate vaccine (PCV7) in children aged 24–59 months who are not completely vaccinated. MMWR Morb Mortal Wkly Rep. 2008;57(13):343–4. PMID: 18385642.

4. Centers for Disease Control and Prevention. Licensure of a 13-valent pneumococcal conjugate vaccine (PCV13) and recommendations for use among children—Advisory Committee on Immunization Practices (ACIP), 2010. MMWR Morb Mortal Wkly Rep. 2010;59(0039):258–61. PMID: 20224542.

5. Schuerman L, Borys D, Hoet B, Forsgren A, Prymula R. Prevention of otitis media: now a reality? Vaccine. 2009;27(42):5748–54. PMID: 19666154.

6. Prymula R, Peeters P, Chrobok V, Kriz P, Novakova E, Kaliskova E, et al. Pneumococcal capsular polysaccharides conjugated to protein D for prevention of acute otitis media caused by both *Streptococcus pneumoniae* and non-typable *Haemophilus influenzae*: a randomised double-blind efficacy study. Lancet. 2006;367(9512):740–8. PMID: 16517274.

7. Block SL, Hedrick J, Harrison CJ, Tyler R, Smith A, Findlay R, et al. Community-wide vaccination with the heptavalent pneumococcal conjugate significantly alters the microbiology of acute otitis media. Pediatr Infect Dis J. 2004;23(9):829–33. PMID: 15361721.

8. Eskola J, Kilpi T, Palmu A, Jokinen J, Haapakoski J, Herva E, et al. Efficacy of a pneumococcal conjugate vaccine against acute otitis media. N Engl J Med. 2001;344(6):403–9. PMID: 11172176.

9. Kilpi T, Ahman H, Jokinen J, Lankinen KS, Palmu A, Savolainen H, et al. Protective efficacy of a second pneumococcal conjugate vaccine against pneumococcal acute otitis media in infants and children: randomized, controlled trial of a 7-valent pneumococcal polysaccharide-meningococcal outer membrane protein complex conjugate vaccine in 1666 children. Clin Infect Dis. 2003;37(9):1155–64. PMID: 14557958.

10. Poehling KA, Szilagyi PG, Grijalva CG, Martin SW, LaFleur B, Mitchel E, et al. Reduction of frequent otitis media and pressure-equalizing tube insertions in children after introduction of pneumococcal conjugate vaccine. Pediatrics. 2007;119(4):707–15. PMID: 17403841.

11. Fletcher MA, Fritzell B. Brief review of the clinical effectiveness of PREVENAR against otitis media. Vaccine. 2007;25(13):2507–12. PMID: 17011085.

12. Dagan R, Frasch C. Clinical characteristics of a novel 10-valent pneumococcal non-typeable *Haemophilus influenzae* protein D conjugate vaccine candidate (PHiD-CV). Introduction. Pediatr Infect Dis J. 2009;28(4 Suppl):S63–5. PMID: 19325448.

13. Prymula R, Hanovcova I, Splino M, Kriz P, Motlova J, Lebedova V, et al. Impact of the 10-valent pneumococcal non-typeable *Haemophilus influenzae* Protein D conjugate vaccine (PHiD-CV) on bacterial nasopharyngeal carriage. Vaccine. 2011;29(10):1959–67. PMID: 21215830.

14. Croxtall JD, Keating GM. Pneumococcal polysaccharide protein D-conjugate vaccine (Synflorix; PHiD-CV). Paediatr Drugs. 2009;11(5):349–57. PMID: 19725600.

15. Hanage WP. Serotype-specific problems associated with pneumococcal conjugate vaccination. Future Microbiol. 2008;3(1):23–30. PMID: 18230031.

16. Pichichero ME. Evolving shifts in otitis media pathogens: relevance to a managed care organization. Am J Manag Care. 2005;11(6 Suppl):S192–201. PMID: 16111442.

17. Coker TR, Chan LS, Newberry SJ, Limbos MA, Suttorp MJ, Shekelle PG, et al. Diagnosis, microbial epidemiology, and antibiotic treatment of acute otitis media in children: a systematic review. JAMA. 2010;304(19):2161–9. PMID: 21081729.

18. Revai K, McCormick DP, Patel J, Grady JJ, Saeed K, Chonmaitree T. Effect of pneumococcal conjugate vaccine on nasopharyngeal bacterial colonization during acute otitis media. Pediatrics. 2006;117(5):1823–9. PMID: 16651345.

19. Hanage WP, Huang SS, Lipsitch M, Bishop CJ, Godoy D, Pelton SI, et al. Diversity and antibiotic resistance among nonvaccine serotypes of *Streptococcus pneumoniae* carriage isolates in the post-heptavalent conjugate vaccine era. J Infect Dis. 2007;195(3):347–52. PMID: 17205472.

20. Kyaw MH, Lynfield R, Schaffner W, Craig AS, Hadler J, Reingold A, et al. Effect of introduction of the pneumococcal conjugate vaccine on drug-resistant *Streptococcus pneumoniae*. N Engl J Med. 2006;354(14):1455–63. PMID: 16598044.

21. Weinberger DM, Malley R, Lipsitch M. Serotype replacement in disease after pneumococcal vaccination. Lancet. 2011;378(9807):1962–73. PMID: 21492929.

22. Tan TQ. Pediatric invasive pneumococcal disease in the United States in the era of pneumococcal conjugate vaccines. Clin Microbiol Rev. 2012;25(3):409–19. PMID: 22763632.

23. Holder RC, Kirse DJ, Evans AK, Peters TR, Poehling KA, Swords WE, et al. One third of middle ear effusions from children undergoing tympanostomy tube placement had multiple bacterial pathogens. BMC Pediatr. 2012;12:87. PMID: 22741759.

24. Pichichero ME, Casey JR, Hoberman A, Schwartz R. Pathogens causing recurrent and difficult-to-treat acute otitis media, 2003–2006. Clin Pediatr (Phila). 2008;47(9):901–6. PMID: 18559884.

25. Berglund J, Vink P, Tavares Da Silva F, Lestrate P, Boutriau D. Safety, immunogenicity, and antibody persistence following an investigational *Streptococcus pneumoniae* and *Haemophilus influenzae* triple-protein vaccine in a phase 1 randomized controlled study in healthy adults. Clin Vaccine Immunol. 2014;21(1):56–65. PMID: 24173029.

26. Palmu A, Jokinen J, Kilpi T. Impact of different case definitions for acute otitis media on the efficacy estimates of a pneumococcal conjugate vaccine. Vaccine. 2008;26(20):2466–70. PMID: 18420315.

27. Murphy TF, Bakaletz LO, Kyd JM, Watson B, Klein DL. Vaccines for otitis media: proposals for overcoming obstacles to progress. Vaccine. 2005;23(21):2696–702. PMID: 15780715.

28. Smith-Vaughan HC, Chang AB, Sarovich DS, Marsh RL, Grimwood K, Leach AJ, et al. Absence of an Important Vaccine and Diagnostic Target in Carriage- and Disease-Related Nontypeable *Haemophilus influenzae*. Clin Vaccine Immunol. 2014;21(2):250–2. PMID: 24285816.

29. Pelton SI, Pettigrew MM, Barenkamp SJ, Godfroid F, Grijalva CG, Leach A, et al. Panel 6: Vaccines. Otolaryngol Head Neck Surg. 2013;148(4 Suppl):E90–101. PMID: 23536534.

30. Marom T, Nokso-Koivisto J, Chonmaitree T. Viral-bacterial interactions in acute otitis media. Curr Allergy Asthma Rep. 2012;12(6):551–8. PMID: 22968233.

31. Rodgers GL, Arguedas A, Cohen R, Dagan R. Global serotype distribution among *Streptococcus pneumoniae* isolates causing otitis media in children: potential implications for pneumococcal conjugate vaccines. Vaccine. 2009;27(29):3802–10. PMID: 19446378.

32. Miyaji EN, Oliveira ML, Carvalho E, Ho PL. Serotype-independent pneumococcal vaccines. Cell Mol Life Sci. 2013;70(18):3303–26. PMID: 23269437.

33. Su YC, Singh B, Riesbeck K. *Moraxella catarrhalis*: from interactions with the host immune system to vaccine development. Future Microbiol. 2012;7(9):1073–100. PMID: 22953708.

34. Smidt M, Battig P, Verhaegh SJ, Niebisch A, Hanner M, Selak S, et al. Comprehensive antigen screening identifies *Moraxella catarrhalis* proteins that induce protection in a mouse pulmonary clearance model. PLoS ONE. 2013;8(5):e64422. PMID: 23671716.

35. Brockson ME, Jurcisek JA, McGillivary G, Bowers MR, Bakaletz LO. Respiratory syncytial virus promotes *Moraxella catarrhalis*-induced ascending experimental otitis media. PLoS ONE. 2012;7(6):e4008. PMID: 22768228.

36. Post JC, Hiller NL, Nistico L, Stoodley P, Ehrlich GD. The role of biofilms in otolaryngologic infections: update 2007. Curr Opin Otolaryngol Head Neck Surg. 2007;15(5):347–51. PMID: 17823552.

37. Post JC, Stoodley P, Hall-Stoodley L, Ehrlich GD. The role of biofilms in otolaryngologic infections. Curr Opin Otolaryngol Head Neck Surg. 2004;12(3):185–90. PMID: 15167027.

38. Slinger R, Chan F, Ferris W, Yeung SW, St Denis M, Gaboury I, et al. Multiple combination antibiotic susceptibility testing of nontypeable *Haemophilus influenzae* biofilms. Diagn Microbiol Infect Dis. 2006;56(3):247–53. PMID: 16769194.

39. Starner TD, Shrout JD, Parsek MR, Appelbaum PC, Kim G. Subinhibitory concentrations of azithromycin decrease nontypeable *Haemophilus influenzae* biofilm formation and diminish established biofilms. Antimicrob Agents Chemother. 2008;52(1):137–45. PMID: 17954687.

40. Kaji C, Watanabe K, Apicella MA, Watanabe H. Antimicrobial effect of fluoroquinolones for the eradication of nontypeable *Haemophilus influenzae* isolates within biofilms. Tohoku J Exp Med. 2008;214(2):121–8. PMID: 18285669.

41. Flemming HC, Wingender J. The biofilm matrix. Nat Rev Microbiol. 2010;8(9):623–33. PMID: 20676145.

42. Rayner MG, Zhang Y, Gorry MC, Chen Y, Post JC, Ehrlich GD. Evidence of bacterial metabolic activity in culture-negative otitis media with effusion. JAMA. 1998;279(4):296–9. PMID: 9450714.

43. Starner TD, Zhang N, Kim G, Apicella MA, McCray PB Jr. *Haemophilus influenzae* forms biofilms on airway epithelia: implications in cystic fibrosis. Am J Respir Crit Care Med. 2006;174(2):213–20. PMID: 16675778.

44. Allegrucci M, Hu FZ, Shen K, Hayes J, Ehrlich GD, Post JC, et al. Phenotypic characterization of *Streptococcus pneumoniae* biofilm development. J Bacteriol. 2006;188(7):2325–35. PMID: 16547018.

45. Pearson MM, Laurence CA, Guinn SE, Hansen EJ. Biofilm formation by *Moraxella catarrhalis in vitro*: roles of the UspA1 adhesin and the Hag hemagglutinin. Infect Immun. 2006;74(3):1588–96. PMID: 16495530.

46. Jurcisek J, Greiner L, Watanabe H, Zaleski A, Apicella MA, Bakaletz LO. Role of sialic acid and complex carbohydrate biosynthesis in biofilm formation by nontypeable *Haemophilus influenzae* in the chinchilla middle ear. Infect Immun. 2005;73(6):3210–8. PMID: 15908345.

47. Murphy TF, Kirkham C. Biofilm formation by nontypeable *Haemophilus influenzae*: strain variability, outer membrane antigen expression and role of pili. BMC Microbiol. 2002;2:7. PMID: 11960553.

48. Hall-Stoodley L, Hu FZ, Gieseke A, Nistico L, Nguyen D, Hayes J, et al. Direct detection of bacterial biofilms on the middle-ear mucosa of children with chronic otitis media. JAMA. 2006;296(2):202–11. PMID: 16835426.

49. Goodman SD, Obergfell KP, Jurcisek JA, Novotny LA, Downey JS, Ayala EA, et al. Biofilms can be dispersed by focusing the immune system on a common family of bacterial nucleoid-associated proteins. Mucosal Immunol. 2011;4(6):625–37. PMID: 21716265.

50. Armbruster CE, Swords WE. Interspecies bacterial communication as a target for therapy in otitis media. Expert Rev Anti Infect Ther. 2010;8(10):1067–70. PMID: 20954869.

51. Daniel M, Chessman R, Al-Zahid S, Richards B, Rahman C, Ashraf W, et al. Biofilm eradication with biodegradable modified-release antibiotic pellets: a potential treatment for glue ear. Arch Otolaryngol Head Neck Surg. 2012;138(10):942–9. PMID: 23069825.

52. Yadav MK, Chae SW, Song JJ. Effect of 5-azacytidine on *in vitro* biofilm formation of *Streptococcus pneumoniae*. Microb Pathog. 2012;53(5–6):219–26. PMID: 22963864.

53. Bakaletz LO. Bacterial biofilms in the upper airway—evidence for role in pathology and implications for treatment of otitis media. Paediatr Respir Rev. 2012;13(3):154–9. PMID: 22726871.

54. Kurola P, Tapiainen T, Sevander J, Kaijalainen T, Leinonen M, Uhari M, et al. Effect of xylitol and other carbon sources on *Streptococcus pneumoniae* biofilm formation and gene expression *in vitro*. APMIS. 2011;119(2):135–42. PMID: 21208281.

55. Hall-Stoodley L, Nistico L, Sambanthamoorthy K, Dice B, Nguyen D, Mershon WJ, et al. Characterization of biofilm matrix, degradation by DNase treatment and evidence of capsule downregulation in *Streptococcus pneumoniae* clinical isolates. BMC Microbiol. 2008;8:173. PMID: 18842140.

56. Centers for Disease Control and Prevention. Recommended immunization schedules for persons aged 0 through 18 years—United States, 2009. MMWR Morb Mortal Wkly Rep. 2009;57(51&52):Q1–4.

57. Prymula R, Chlibek R, Splino M, Kaliskova E, Kohl I, Lommel P, et al. Safety of the 11-valent pneumococcal vaccine conjugated to non-typeable *Haemophilus influenzae*-derived protein D in the first 2 years of life and immunogenicity of the co-administered hexavalent diphtheria, tetanus, acellular pertussis, hepatitis B, inactivated polio virus, *Haemophilus influenzae* type b and control hepatitis A vaccines. Vaccine. 2008;26(35):4563–70. PMID: 18602724.

58. Koslap-Petraco MB, Parsons T. Communicating the benefits of combination vaccines to parents and health care providers. J Pediatr Health Care. 2003;17(2):53–7. PMID: 12665726.

59. Kurstak E. New vaccines development, immunisation and immunotherapy. Vaccine. 2007;25(16):2960–2. PMID: 17316930.

60. De Magistris MT. Mucosal delivery of vaccine antigens and its advantages in pediatrics. Adv Drug Deliv Rev. 2006;58(1):52–67. PMID: 16516335.

61. Kersten G, Hirschberg H. Needle-free vaccine delivery. Expert Opin Drug Deliv. 2007;4(5):459–74. PMID: 17880271.

62. Levine MM. Can needle-free administration of vaccines become the norm in global immunization? Nat Med. 2003;9(1):99–103. PMID: 12514720.

63. Silin DS, Lyubomska OV, Jirathitikal V, Bourinbaiar AS. Oral vaccination: where we are? Expert Opin Drug Deliv. 2007;4(4):323–40. PMID: 17683247.

64. Ostberg KL, Russell MW, Murphy TF. Mucosal immunization of mice with recombinant OMP P2 induces antibodies that bind to surface epitopes of multiple strains of nontypeable *Haemophilus influenzae*. Mucosal Immunol. 2009;2(1):63–73. PMID: 19079335.

65. Sabirov A, Metzger DW. Mouse models for the study of mucosal vaccination against otitis media. Vaccine. 2008;26(12):1501–24. PMID: 18295938.

66. Novotny LA, Clements JD, Bakaletz LO. Kinetic analysis and evaluation of the mechanisms involved in the resolution of experimental nontypeable *Haemophilus influenzae*-induced otitis media after transcutaneous immunization. Vaccine. 2013;31(34):3417–26. PMID: 23092856.

67. Novotny LA, Clements JD, Bakaletz LO. Transcutaneous immunization as preventative and therapeutic regimens to protect against experimental otitis media due to nontypeable *Haemophilus influenzae*. Mucosal Immunol. 2011;4(4):456–67. PMID: 21326197.

68. Prevention of hearing impairment from chronic otitis media. WHO/CIBA Foundation Workshop. London: The CIBA Foundation; 1996, 19–21 November 1996.

69. Di Francesco RC, Sampaio PL, Bento RF. Correlation between otitis media and craniofacial morphology in adults. Ear Nose Throat J. 2007;86(12):738–43. PMID: 18217377.

70. Singleton RJ, Holman RC, Plant R, Yorita KL, Holve S, Paisano EL, et al. Trends in otitis media and myringtomy with tube placement among American Indian/Alaska native children and the US general population of children. Pediatr Infect Dis J. 2009;28(2):102–7. PMID: 19131901.

71. Akira S. Toll-like receptors: lessons from knockout mice. Biochem Soc Trans. 2000;28(5):551–6. PMID: 11044373.

72. Cassell GH, Archer GL, Beam TR, Gilchrist MJ, Goldmann D, Hooper DC, et al. Report of the ASM Task Force on Antibiotic Resistance. July 6, 1994, 1994; Washington D.C.

73. Infante-Rivard C, Fernandez A. Otitis media in children: frequency, risk factors, and research avenues. Epidemiol Rev. 1993;15(2):444–65. PMID: 8174666.

74. Stool SE, Berg AO, Berman S, Carney CJ, Cooley JR, Culpepper L, et al. Otitis Media with Effusion in Young Children. Clinical Practice Guideline. Rockville: Agency for Health Care Policy and Research, Public Health Service, U.S. Department of Health and Human Services; 1994.

75. Ahmed S, Shapiro NL, Bhattacharyya N. Incremental health care utilization and costs for acute otitis media in children. Laryngoscope. 2014;124(1):301–5. PMID: 23649905.

76. Pichichero ME. Otitis media. Pediatr Clin North Am. 2013;60(2):391–407. PMID: 23481107.

77. Monasta L, Ronfani L, Marchetti F, Montico M, Vecchi Brumatti L, Bavcar A, et al. Burden of disease caused by otitis media: systematic review and global estimates. PLoS ONE. 2012;7(4):e36226. PMID: 22558393.

78. American Academy of Pediatrics Subcommittee on Management of Acute Otitis Media. Diagnosis and management of acute otitis media. Pediatrics. 2004;113(5):1451–65. PMID: 15121972.

79. Acuin J, Department of Child and Adolescent Health and Development, Team for Prevention of Blindness and Deafness, The World Health Organization.

Chronic suppurative otitis media: burden of illness and management options; 2004. http://www.who.int/pbd/publications/Chronicsuppurativeotitis_media.pdf.

80. Baldwin RL. Effects of otitis media on child development. Am J Otol. 1993;14(6):601–4. PMID: 7507647.

81. Johnson DL, McCormick DP, Baldwin CD. Early middle ear effusion and language at age seven. J Commun Disord. 2008;41(1):20–32. PMID: 17418231.

82. McCormick DP, Johnson DL, Baldwin CD. Early middle ear effusion and school achievement at age seven years. Ambul Pediatr. 2006;6(5):280–7. PMID: 17000418.

83. Hunter LL, Margolis RH, Giebink GS. Identification of hearing loss in children with otitis media. Ann Otol Rhinol Laryngol Suppl. 1994;163:59–61. PMID: 8179273.

84. Li JD, Hermansson A, Ryan AF, Bakaletz LO, Brown SD, Cheeseman MT, et al. Panel 4: recent advances in otitis media in molecular biology, biochemistry, genetics, and animal models. Otolaryngol Head Neck Surg. 2013;148(4 Suppl):E52-63. PMID: 23536532.

85. Venekamp RP, Sanders S, Glasziou PP, Del Mar CB, Rovers MM. Antibiotics for acute otitis media in children. Cochrane Database Syst Rev. 2013;1:CD000219. PMID: 23440776.

86. Song JH, Dagan R, Klugman KP, Fritzell B. The relationship between pneumococcal serotypes and antibiotic resistance. Vaccine. 2012;30(17):2728–37. PMID: 22330126.

87. Leibovitz E, Broides A, Greenberg D, Newman N. Current management of pediatric acute otitis media. Expert Rev Anti Infect Ther. 2010;8(2):151–61. PMID: 20109045.

88. Wang EE, Einarson TR, Kellner JD, Conly JM. Antibiotic prescribing for Canadian preschool children: evidence of overprescribing for viral respiratory infections. Clin Infect Dis. 1999;29(1):155–60. PMID: 10433579.

89. Berman S, Roard R, PA-C M, Luckey C. Theoretical cost effectiveness of management options for children with persisting middle ear effusions. Pediatrics. 1994;93(3):353–63. PMID: 8115191.

90. Bright RA, Moore RM Jr, Jeng LL, Sharkness CM, Hamburger SE, Hamilton PM. The prevalence of tympanostomy tubes in children in the United States, 1988. Am J Public Health. 1993;83(7):1026–8. PMID: 8328599.

91. Cimons M. Watchful Waiting Advised When Treating Otitis Media. ASM News. 1994;60:527–8..

92. Paap CM. Management of otitis media with effusion in young children. Ann Pharmacother. 1996;30(11):1291–7. PMID: 8913412.

93. O'Brien MA, Prosser LA, Paradise JL, Ray GT, Kulldorff M, Kurs-Lasky M, et al. New vaccines against otitis media: projected benefits and cost-effectiveness. Pediatrics. 2009;123(6):1452–63. PMID: 19482754.

94. Alsarraf R, Jung CJ, Perkins J, Crowley C, Alsarraf NW, Gates GA. Measuring the indirect and direct costs of acute otitis media. Arch Otolaryngol Head Neck Surg. 1999;125(1):12–8. PMID: 9932581..

95. Cassell GH. New and reemerging infectious diseases, a global crisis and immediate threat to the nation's health, the role of research. Washington, D.C.: American Society for Microbiology; 1997.

96. Kaplan B, Wandstrat TL, Cunningham JR. Overall cost in the treatment of otitis media. Pediatr Infect Dis J. 1997;16(2 Suppl):S9-11. PMID: 9041621.

97. Vergison A, Dagan R, Arguedas A, Bonhoeffer J, Cohen R, Dhooge I, et al. Otitis media and its consequences: beyond the earache. Lancet Infect Dis. 2010;10(3):195–203. PMID: 20185098.

Antibiotics for Otitis Media: To Treat or Not to Treat

10

Jill Arganbright, Amanda G. Ruiz and Peggy Kelley

Introduction

Otitis media (OM) is one of the most common diseases of early infancy and childhood [1]. By age 3, approximately 85 % of children will have experienced at least one episode of acute otitis media (AOM). OM is also the most common diagnosis for which antibiotics are prescribed to children [2]; in fact, AOM accounts for 60 % of all antibiotics written for children [3]. As such the societal cost of this disease is vast; with $ 5.3 billion of direct and indirect costs is attributed to the diagnosis and treatment of pediatric OM [4]. Despite numerous studies, antibiotic treatment of OM has historically been controversial [5]. Recently published clinical practice guidelines for the treatment of AOM in 2013, [6] otitis media with effusion (OME) in 2004, [7], and tympanostomy tubes (TT) in children in 2014 [8] have provided updated evidence-based recommendations for clinicians and provide a starting point for standardization of management of this common entity. The goal of this chapter is to use the published guidelines and current literature to highlight when treatment with antibiotic therapy is indicated for specific OM disease processes: AOM, chronic OME, chronic suppurative otitis media, and AOM when TT is present.

Acute Otitis Media

The 2013 Guidelines [6] for the treatment of AOM define "severe AOM" as AOM with the presence of moderate to severe otalgia or fever equal or higher than 39.0 °C. The definition for "non-severe" AOM is AOM with the presence of mild otalgia and temperature below 39.0 °C. The guidelines recommend clinicians prescribe antibiotic therapy for bilateral AOM in children younger than 2 years old, children 6 months and older with evidence of severe AOM (bilateral or unilateral), and to all patients with otorrhea. The recommendations state for patients 6 months to 2 years with non-severe unilateral AOM, or patients older than 2 years with bilateral non-severe AOM without otorrhea, clinicians should prescribe antibiotic therapy or offer observation with close follow-up (48–72 h) based on joint decision-making with the parents and caregivers.

Benefits of Antibiotics for Non-severe AOM Although rare, the fear of complications (i.e., mastoiditis and meningitis) has been a driving force for the treatment of AOM with antibiotics. In addition, studies have shown patients receiving antibiotics at the time of AOM have a quicker resolution of symptoms compared to those patients not receiving antibiotics [3].

P. Kelley (✉)
Otolaryngology, Children's Hospital Colorado,
13123 E. 16th Ave B-455, Aurora, CO 80045, USA
e-mail: peggy.kelley@childrenscolorado.org

J. Arganbright
Otolaryngology, Children's Mercy Hospital and Clinics,
2401 Gillham Road, Kansas City, MO 64108, USA
e-mail: jarganbright@cmh.edu

A. G. Ruiz
Otolaryngology, The University of Colorado
School of Medicine, Children's Hospital Colorado,
13123 East 16th, Box 455, Aurora, CO 80045, USA
e-mail: amanda.ruiz@childrenscolorado.org

© Springer International Publishing Switzerland 2015
D. Preciado (ed.), *Otitis Media: State of the art concepts and treatment*, DOI 10.1007/978-3-319-17888-2_10

Although this has been described as a rather small treatment effect difference, it is important to consider the improvement in the quality of life the rapidity of symptom resolution may provide—including parent anxiety with the continuation of symptoms, the economic implications of parents' need to take additional time off work to care for their sick child and/or additional doctor visits, as well as extended number of missed school days for the child [3]. A study by Meopol et al. [9] estimated the economic cost that deferring one antibiotic course for a child meeting the current US guidelines for AOM treatment would result in 0.3–4 lost quality-adjusted life-days, which may not be as desirable from a parental perspective.

Benefits of the "Watchful Waiting" Method for Non-severe AOM With the emergence of multibacterial drug-resistant bacteria [10] as well as other known adverse effects of antibiotics including medication side effects (rash, diarrhea, vomiting, and fungal infection) and treatment cost, the therapeutic approach to treating AOM has been debated [11]. A randomized controlled trial compared patients diagnosed with AOM who were placed immediately on antibiotics to those placed in a "watchful waiting" (WW) group. The reported 66 % of patients in the WW group improved without antibiotic therapy. Treatment failures did not vary with age. Parent satisfaction was the same between the WW and antibiotic group. Immediate antibiotic treatment was associated with decreased number of treatment failures, but had increased antibiotic-related adverse events [12].

A study from the Netherlands [13] reported 4860 consecutive Dutch patients (<2 years old) with AOM who were treated with nose drops and analgesic alone. They report 90 % recovered within the first few days and concluded that AOM in children can be treated symptomatically without antibiotic therapy for the first 3–4 days; of note, despite the lack of antibiotic therapy, this study had only one new case of mastoiditis and no cases of bacterial meningitis.

Highlighting the difficulty of clinically implementing new guidelines, three studies looked US physicians treatment of AOM after guidelines [6] were released and found the management of AOM without antibiotics had not increased [14] and the variability of prescribed antibiotics for AOM actually increased from before the published guideline recommendations [15]. Chu et al. looked retrospectively at 207 patients treated for uncomplicated AOM and found overall adherence to the guidelines was only 8.2 % [16].

The decision to proceed with the WW method is multifactorial and does require a trusted physician–parent/patient relationship. McCormick et al. [12] describe five key factors needed in implementing a WW strategy: a method to classify AOM severity, parent education regarding the risks and benefits of treatment, management of AOM symptoms, access to follow-up care, and use of an effective antibiotic regimen if needed. When considering the WW method, it is important to take into consideration the patient's age, degree of certainty about the diagnosis, the severity of the illness, as well as parental concerns/level of comfort.

Antibiotic Selection When the decision has been made to treat AOM with an antibiotic, clinical guidelines recommend amoxicillin (80–90 mg/kg/day in two divided doses) in the event the patient has not received amoxicillin within the prior 30 days and is not allergic to penicillin [6]. If the patient has been treated with amoxicillin within 30 days or if the patient has a history of recurrent AOM unresponsive to amoxicillin, high-dose amoxicillin–clavulanate (90 mg/kg/day divided into two doses) should be prescribed. Patient reassessment to evaluate whether a change in antibiotic therapy is indicated should occur if the child's symptoms have worsened or failed to respond to the initial antibiotic treatment within 48–72 h. Prophylactic antibioticsto prevent AOM are not recommended [6].

Chronic Suppurative Otitis Media

Chronic suppurative otitis media (CSOM) is defined as a chronic infection of the middle ear in which a non-intact tympanic membrane and otorrhea are present [17]. There is no consensus on the duration of otorrhea required to make the diagnosis, although the World Health Organization uses a definition where the otorrhea must be present for "at least 2 weeks," [18] while others define "chronic" as a persistence of symptoms for 6 weeks or greater [19–21]. CSOM remains one of the most common chronic infections of childhood in many developing countries [22]. Sequela of CSOM can include chronic hearing loss and subsequent speech/language delay, as well as the potential danger of life-threatening suppurative complications (i.e., mastoiditis, meningitis, and epidural abscess).

An Optimal treatment strategy has not yet been established but topical treatment with otic antibiotic drops, combined with frequent and aggressive aural toilet have been the mainstay [21, 23, 24]. The effectiveness of ototopical drops was evaluated in a Cochrane Review [23] which concluded that antibiotic or antiseptic eardrops accompanied by aural toilet was the most effective treatment; this treatment regimen was more effective than systemic antibiotics, and aural toilet alone. Combined topical and systemic antibiotics were not more effective than treatment with topical antibiotics alone in terms of otorrhea resolution. Several studies have supported quinolone eardrops to be more effective than non-quinolones [18, 23, 25, 26]. When granulation tissue is present, adding a steroid to the ototopical antibiotics is recommended [21, 24].

Consensus is lacking regarding the utility of systemic antibiotics for this disease process. An expert panel by the American Academy of Otolaryngology-Head and Neck Surgery concluded in the absence of systemic infections or serious underlying disease, topical antibiotics alone should be considered first-line treatment [24]. Evidence is also lacking regarding choice of antibiotic and duration of therapy; both broad-spectrum antibiotics as well as culture-directed therapy have been advocated as initial oral therapy for CSOM [22]. Finally, in children with evidence of complications of CSOM may require CT scan and initiation of intravenous antibiotics [19, 20, 25].

Chronic Otitis Media with Effusion

OME is the most common cause of childhood hearing loss [27]. Several studies have looked at whether there is benefit of medical therapy for persistent OME. Although some studies report a statistically significant benefit when using specific medications [28, 29], these are short-term benefits and relatively small in overall magnitude. In a meta-analysis by Williams et al. [28], they found six patients needed to be treated to improve the short-term outcome in one patient. The authors' question the utility of this short-term benefit given the major goal of treatment of OME is the prevention of language or developmental delays second to hearing loss, which occur over a long period of time. This study also found no significant difference between placebo and antibiotics in eight studies of long-term outcomes of OME [28]. The 2004 clinical guidelines [7] report the risk of adverse events which may occur with all medical therapies, outweigh the small benefit they may provide, and do not recommend antibiotics. A Cochrane Review published in 2012 [30] does not support the routine use of antibiotics for children with OME. In the review, the largest clinical improvement was found in children treated with continuous antibiotics for 4 weeks to 3 months. The authors' conclude that the modest benefit of antibiotic therapy observed must be balanced against the risks of adverse effects of antibiotics and the emergence of bacterial resistance.

Adjuvant Therapy for OME The use of antihistamines and decongestants as adjuvants in the treatment of OME has not been shown to be of significant clinical benefit [31, 32]. The 2004 clinical guidelines [7] also do not recommend antihistamines and decongestants. Oral steroid therapy is not recommended, highlighting the extensive side effect profile of oral steroids compared to the short-term benefit it may produce [7]. Intranasal steroids are known to have less systemic absorption and thus fewer adverse effects; however, a Cochrane Review published in 2010 found no evidence of benefit from the treatment of OME with topical intranasal steroids, alone or in combination with an antibiotic either at short-term or longer term follow-up [33].

Acute Otitis Media with Tympanostomy Tubes

Otorrhea is the most common sequela of TT, with a mean incidence estimated between 5 and 20%, but has been reported as high as 83% with prospective surveillance [8, 24].

The most common cause of tympanostomy tube otorrhea is AOM [34]. Clinical practice guidelines published in 2013 [8] recommend clinicians prescribe topical antibiotic ear drops only, without oral antibiotics, for children with uncomplicated, acute (less than 4 weeks) tympanostomy tube otorrhea. In support of these recommendation is a study by van Dongen et al. published in 2014 in the *New England Journal of Medicine* randomly assigned 230 children with acute tympanostomy tube otorrhea to receive either topical antibiotic-glucocorticoid eardrops or oral amoxicillin–clavulanate (Augmentin) suspension. They concluded the eardrops were more effective than oral antibiotics and no complications of OM were reported [35]. Goldblatt et al. [36] published a multicenter, randomized controlled trial of systemic antibiotic (Augmentin) versus topical ofloxacin in the treatment of AOM in children with TT after concluded topical ofloxacin was as effective and better tolerated than Augmentin. Another study compared ciprofloxacin-dexamethasone drops to oral Augmentin; this multicenter randomized controlled trial concluded the topical treatment resulted in a significant reduction in duration of otorrhea and significantly improved cure rate with less adverse effects than the oral antibiotic [37].

Roland et al published a multicenter randomized controlled trial comparing topical antibiotic with steroid (ciprofloxacin-dexamethasone) to topical antibiotic alone (ciprofloxacin), and found the group with topical antibiotic and steroid had significantly fewer treatment failures, reduced median time to cessation of otorrhea,

and greater eradication of pathogens [38]. The benefits gained when adding dexamethasone to a topical antibiotic need to be balanced with the increase in treatment cost [34].

The treatment guidelines [8] do recommend systemic antibiotic therapy with or without concurrent topical antibiotic therapy when the following are present: cellulitis of the pinna or adjacent skin, concurrent bacterial infection (i.e., strep pharyngitis and sinusitis), toxic appearance and high fevers, otorrhea persists or worsens despite topical antibiotic therapy, administration of ear drops is not possible second to discomfort and child intolerance, patient is in an immunocompromised state, or cost limitations prevent access to non-ototoxic topical antibiotic drops. Studies show 4–8% of children treated with topical otic drops will require oral antibiotic therapy for persistent symptoms [8]. Additional considerations when a child has failed topical quinolone otic drops include evaluation of ear tube for possible blockage and culture of the persistent drainage.

Conclusion

OM is an extremely common diagnosis in children for which historically treatment recommendations have varied immensely. Recently, evidence-based clinical guidelines have been introduced to assist practitioners by providing guidance in treatment recommendations and indications for antibiotic usage. Future research must continue to strengthen or refute the evidence behind the current recommendations as well as better define recommendations for entities such as CSOM where treatment regiments are still being established.

References

1. Wolleswinkel-van den Bosch JH, Stolk EA, Francois M, Gasparini R, Brosa M. The health care burden and societal impact of acute otitis media in seven European countries: results of an Internet survey. Vaccine. 2010;28(6):G39–52. doi:10.1016/j.vaccine.2010.06.014.

2. Grossman Z, Silverman BG, Miron D. Physician specialty is associated with adherence to treatment guidelines for acute otitis media in children. Acta Paediatr. 2013;102(1):e29–33. doi:10.1111/apa.12051.

3. Vouloumanou EK, Karageorgopoulos DE, Kazantzi MS, Kapaskelis AM, Falagas ME. Antibiotics versus placebo or watchful waiting for acute otitis media: a meta-analysis of randomized controlled trials. J Antimicrob Chemother. 2009;64(1):16–24. doi:10.1093/jac/dkp166.

4. Montgomery D. A new approach to treating acute otitis media. J Pediatr Health Care. 2005;19(1):50–2.

5. Elden LM, Spiro DM. Acute otitis media-to treat or not to treat? Pediatr Emerg Care. 2006;22(4):283–6.

6. Lieberthal AS, Carroll AE, Chonmaitree T, et al. The diagnosis and management of acute otitis media. Pediatrics. 2013;131(3):e964–99. doi:10.1542/peds.2012-3488.

7. Rosenfeld RM, Culpepper L, Doyle KJ, et al. Clinical practice guideline: otitis media with effusion. Otolaryngol Head Neck Surg. 2004;130(5):95–118.

8. Rosenfeld RM, Schwartz SR, Pynnonen MA, et al. Clinical practice guideline: tympanostomy tubes in children. Otolaryngol Head Neck Surg. 2013;149(1):1–35.doi:10.1177/0194599813487302.

9. Meropol SB. Valuing reduced antibiotic use for pediatric acute otitis media. Pediatrics. 2008;121(4):669–73. doi:10.1542/peds.2007-1914.

10. Sagraves R. Increasing antibiotic resistance: its effect on the therapy for otitis media. J Pediatr Health Care. 2002;16(2):79–85.

11. Stevanovic T, Komazec Z, Lemajic-Komazec S, Jovic R. Acute otitis media: to follow-up or treat? Int J Pediatr Otorhinolaryngol. 2010;74(8):930–3. doi:10.1016/j.ijporl.2010.05.017.

12. McCormick DP, Chonmaitree T, Pittman C, et al. Nonsevere acute otitis media: a clinical trial comparing outcomes of watchful waiting versus immediate antibiotic treatment. Pediatrics. 2005;115(6):1455–65.

13. van Buchem FL, Peeters MF, van't Hof MA. Acute otitis media: a new treatment strategy. Br Med J (Clin Res Ed). 1985;290(6474):1033–7.

14. Coco A, Vernacchio L, Horst M, Anderson A. Management of acute otitis media after publication of the 2004 AAP and AAFP clinical practice guideline. Pediatrics. 2010;125(2):214–20. doi:10.1542/peds.2009-1115.

15. Vernacchio L, Vezina RM, Mitchell AA. Management of acute otitis media by primary care physicians: trends since the release of the 2004 American Academy of Pediatrics/American Academy of Family Physicians clinical practice guideline. Pediatrics. 2007;120(2):281–7.

16. Chu CH, Wang MC, Lin LY, Shiao AS. Physicians are not adherent to clinical practice guidelines for acute otitis media. Int J Pediatr Otorhinolaryngol. 2011;75(7):955–9.doi:10.1016/j.ijporl.2011.04.019.

17. Bluestone CD. Epidemiology and pathogenesis of chronic suppurative otitis media: implications for prevention and treatment. Int J Pediatr Otorhinolaryngol. 1998;42(3):207–23.

18. Woodfield G, Dugdale A. Evidence behind the WHO guidelines: hospital care for children: what is the most effective antibiotic regime for chronic suppurative otitis media in children? J Trop Pediatr. 2008;54(3):151–6. doi:10.1093/tropej/fmn042.

19. Kenna MA, Rosane BA, Bluestone CD. Medical management of chronic suppurative otitis media without cholesteatoma in children—update 1992. Am J Otol. 1993;14(5):469–73.

20. Fliss DM, Dagan R, Houri Z, Leiberman A. Medical management of chronic suppurative otitis media without cholesteatoma in children. J Pediatr. 1990;116(6):991–6.

21. Roland PS. Chronic suppurative otitis media: a clinical overview. Ear Nose Throat J. 2002;81(8):8–10.

22. Verhoeff M, van der Veen EL, Rovers MM, Sanders EA, Schilder AG. Chronic suppurative otitis media: a review. Int J Pediatr Otorhinolaryngol. 2006;70(1):1–12.

23. Acuin J, Smith A, Mackenzie I. Interventions for chronic suppurative otitis media. Cochrane Database Syst Rev. 2000;(2):CD000473. Review. Update in: Cochrane Database Syst Rev. 1998;(4):CD000473. PubMed PMID: 10796720.

24. Hannley MT, Denneny JC, 3rd, Holzer SS. Use of ototopical antibiotics in treating 3 common ear diseases. Otolaryngol Head Neck Surg. 2000;122(6):934–40.

25. Abes G, Espallardo N, Tong M, et al. A systematic review of the effectiveness of ofloxaxin otic solution for the treatment of suppurative otitis media. ORL J Otorhinolaryngol Relat Spec. 2003;65(2):106–16.

26. Arguedas A, Loaiza C, Herrera JF, Mohs E. Antimicrobial therapy for children with chronic suppurative otitis media without cholesteatoma. Pediatr Infect Dis J. 1994;13(10):878–82.

27. Robb PJ, Williamson I. Otitis media with effusion in children: current management. J Paediatr Child Health. 2011;22(1):9–12.

28. Williams RL, Chalmers TC, Stange KC, Chalmers FT, Bowlin SJ. Use of antibiotics in preventing recurrent acute otitis media and in treating otitis media with effusion. A meta-analytic attempt to resolve the brouhaha. JAMA. 1993;270(11):1344–51.

29. Rosenfeld RM, Post JC. Meta-analysis of antibiotics for the treatment of otitis media with effusion. Otolaryngol Head Neck Surg. 1992;106(4):378–86.

30. van Zon A, van der Heijden GJ, van Dongen TM, Burton MJ, Schilder AG. Antibiotics for otitis media with effusion in children. Cochrane Database Syst Rev. 2012;9:CD009163. doi:10.1002/14651858.CD009163.pub2.

31. Bonney AG, Goldman RD. Antihistamines for children with otitis media. Can Fam Physician. 2014;60(1):43–6.

32. Choung YH, Shin YR, Choi SJ, et al. Management for the children with otitis media with effusion in the tertiary hospital. Clin Exp Otorhinolaryngol. 2008;1(4):201–5. doi:10.3342/ceo.2008.1.4.201.

33. Simpson SA, Lewis R, van der Voort J, Butler CC. Oral or topical nasal steroids for hearing loss associated with otitis media with effusion in children. Cochrane Database Syst Rev. 2011;(5):CD001935. doi:10.1002/14651858.CD001935.pub3.

34. Schmelzle J, Birtwhistle RV, Tan AK. Acute otitis media in children with tympanostomy tubes. Can Fam Physician. 2008;54(8):1123–7.

35. van Dongen TM, van der Heijden GJ, Venekamp RP, Rovers MM, Schilder AG. A trial of treatment for acute otorrhea in children with tympanostomy tubes. N Engl J Med. 2014;370(8):723–33.

36. Goldblatt EL, Dohar J, Nozza RJ, et al. Topical ofloxacin versus systemic amoxicillin/clavulanate in purulent otorrhea in children with tympanostomy tubes. Int J Pediatr Otorhinolaryngol. 1998;46(1–2):91–101.

37. Dohar J, Giles W, Roland P, et al. Topical ciprofloxacin/dexamethasone superior to oral amoxicillin/clavulanic acid in acute otitis media with otorrhea through tympanostomy tubes. Pediatrics. 2006;118(3):e561–9.

38. Roland PS, Anon JB, Moe RD, et al. Topical ciprofloxacin/dexamethasone is superior to ciprofloxacin alone in pediatric patients with acute otitis media and otorrhea through tympanostomy tubes. Laryngoscope. 2003;113(12):2116–22.

Tympanostomy Tube Placement for Management of Otitis Media

11

Lyndy Wilcox and Craig Derkay

Introduction

Otitis media (OM) is defined as inflammation of the middle ear (ME). It can be subclassified into two main groups: acute otitis media (AOM) and otitis media with effusion (OME). OME indicates the presence of a middle ear effusion (MEE), which can subsequently cause conductive hearing loss (CHL), disequilibrium, and tinnitus. OME is considered chronic if the effusion lasts for 3 or more months. AOM, on the other hand, is distinguished by signs and symptoms of infection, such as bulging and erythema of the tympanic membrane (TM), fever, and otalgia, in addition to an MEE. AOM can be further classified as recurrent or persistent. A child who has three or more episodes in 6 months or four episodes in a 12-month period with at least one episode in the past 6 months can be considered to have recurrent AOM (RAOM), whereas a child with an episode of AOM that persists during antimicrobial therapy or relapses within 1 month of completing appropriate antibiotic therapy may be considered to have persistent AOM [1].

Epidemiology

Children under the age of 7 are at the highest risk for OM with a high incidence in this age group [2]. By 3 years of age, most children have had at least one episode of AOM, and nearly 40 % have had three or more infections by 6 years of age [3]. More than 50 % of children have an episode of OME before their first birthday with more than 60 % developing OME before age 2 [4, 5]. It is estimated that 90 % of children will have at least one episode of OM by the age of 10 years [6].

OM accounts for 14–18 % of ambulatory care visits in children under the age of 4 years [7] and for 17.6 % of all visits to otolaryngologists [8]. This translates into AOM and, unfortunately, OME being the most common indication for antibiotic prescription in children [9, 10]. OME and RAOM are also the most common indications for tympanostomy tube (TT) placement in children [11] as they can prevent and relieve fluid accumulation, decrease the rate of recurrent infections, provide a conduit for drainage and administration of topical antibiotics, improve hearing, and improve quality of life (QOL) [12, 13]. Consequently, placement of TTs is the most common surgery performed in the pediatric population with almost 670,000 children undergoing the procedure each year [14]. Bilateral myringotomy with TT (BMTT) placement accounts for more than 20 % of all ambulatory surgeries in children, and by age 3 years, as many as 1 in 15 children (6.8 %) will have undergone the procedure

C. Derkay (✉) · L. Wilcox
Department of Otolaryngology Head Neck Surgery,
Eastern Virginia Medical School, Children's Hospital
of the King's Daughters, 601 Children's Lane, 2nd Floor,
Norfolk, VA 23507, USA
e-mail: craig.derkay@chkd.org

© Springer International Publishing Switzerland 2015
D. Preciado (ed.), *Otitis Media: State of the art concepts and treatment*, DOI 10.1007/978-3-319-17888-2_11

[1]. The annual cost of the medical and surgical therapy for the disease in the USA is estimated at $ 4–5 billion for children under 5 years of age [5, 10, 15].This financial burden includes not only the direct costs of doctor's visits, testing, medical treatment, and surgical therapy but also the indirect costs of child absence from school and missed days of work for parents. Additionally, the emotional and social burden of the disease and its long-term impact should be considered. Despite the prevalence of OM and the frequency of insertion of TT, only recently have guidelines regarding their use been developed.

Evaluation for Tympanostomy Tube Placement

When children are referred for evaluation for BMTT, the history should include number of distinct episodes of AOM, the severity and duration of these episodes, antibiotics or other treatments prescribed and their benefits, adverse drug reactions or complications that have occurred as part of the episodes, and the persistence of OME after episodes of AOM. Age at first AOM and the timing of the most recent infection prior to visiting the otolaryngologist are additional helpful pieces of the history to elicit. Typically, OME can be expected to clear within 1 month of antibiotic treatment in 60 % of children with AOM and by 3 months in about 90 % of children [16]. OME not related to AOM is less likely to resolve spontaneously with resolution rates ranging from 28 to 52 % after 3 or 4 months [17, 18]. If OME fails to clear after 3 months, it is considered chronic OME and may require further treatment. Any concerns of hearing loss (HL) or speech delay should be elicited. Caregivers should be questioned regarding the results of the child's newborn hearing screening. Other comorbidities that could complicate management of the child's ME disease, such as Down syndrome, attention deficit hyperactivity disorders, autism, learning disabilities, premature birth, cerebral palsy, seizure disorders, asthma, and sickle cell disease, should be identified. Modifiable environmental influences, such as daycare attendance with more than 5 unrelated children, pacifier use after age 2, and secondhand smoke exposure, should be discussed. Past medical history, prior surgeries on the head and neck, and parental or sibling history of otolaryngology procedures may also provide important details aiding the clinician to develop a treatment plan with the child's caregivers.

The gold standard for diagnosis of AOM and OME is pneumatic otoscopy. The exam in AOM reveals an opaque, bulging, and intensely erythematous TM with decreased mobility with suppurative MEE. Moderate to severe bulging of the TM has been shown to be the finding most predictive of AOM. The symptoms should be seen in conjunction with a recent onset of otalgia to confirm the diagnosis. Conversely, a diagnosis of AOM should not be made without the presence of an MEE [19]. In OME, pneumatic otoscopy will also reveal an MEE with decreased mobility of the TM, often with a yellow or orange-colored serous fluid visible, as opposed to the opaque fluid behind an inflamed TM in AOM. The TM is usually retracted or in a neutral position (vs. bulging) in OME. Children with a history of frequent infections may develop myringosclerosis, atelectasis or retraction pockets, and perforations of the TM [20]. The physical examination should also be directed to discovering anomalies that may contribute to ME disease such as the presence of a cleft palate, submucous cleft palate, bifid uvula, "adenoid facies," or "allergic shiners". Additional testing in children with OM being considered for surgical therapy of their ME disease should include tympanometry and audiometry. These studies are often normal between episodes in a child with RAOM; however, a child with chronic OME would be expected to have a flat (type B) tympanogram with normal canal volume along with some degree of CHL, typically at least seen in the low frequencies. Current guidelines recommend obtaining an age-appropriate hearing test on all children with OME of less than 3 months duration prior to surgical intervention [1]. This allows documentation of hearing status with a baseline prior to surgical intervention. The average HL in children with OME is 28 dB but can exceed 35 dB in 20 % of cases [21, 22]. The hearing test may provide the surgeon with additional information on which to base operative decisions or detect coexisting sensorineural hearing loss (SNHL).

The determination of children with RAOM or chronic otitis media with effusion (COME) who are "at-risk" for speech, language, or learning problems from their ear disease due to baseline sensory, physical, cognitive, or behavioral factors is also important in determining the most appropriate management [1]. For example, children with SNHL, autistic spectrum disorders, low birth weight, craniofacial or other genetic syndromes, cerebral palsy, blindness, and cleft palates may be at even greater risk of experiencing further delays in their communication skills if they also suffer from additional issues with their hearing related to OME or AOM. While most high-quality studies exclude this population of children, they are widely assumed to be less tolerant of OME or RAOM [23, 24].

Treatment

Surgical Tympanostomy Tube Placement Guidelines

Surgical As previously noted, BMTT is the most common surgical procedure performed in the pediatric population. Guidelines for BMTT in children aged 6 months to 12 years were released in July of 2013 providing long-awaited recommendations to address patient selection, surgical indications for, and management of TTs [1]. The guidelines recommend the following indications for performing BMTT:

1. *BMTT should not be performed in children with a single episode of OME of less than 3 months duration, except in "at-risk" children*[1]. This recommendation is based on the natural history of OME [3, 16], and it aims to avoid surgery for a condition with a high likelihood of spontaneous resolution within 3 months.

2. *Children with bilateral COME of less than 3 months duration and documented hearing difficulties, not necessarily HL, should be offered BMTT* [1]. This recommendation is based on multiple randomized controlled trials (RCTs) showing significant benefits to BMTT in this situation. These benefits include reduced prevalence of MEE, improved hearing, and improved QOL for both the patient and the caregiver [25, 26]. Also, unlike OME of less than 3 months duration, there is a low likelihood of resolution of fluid after 3 months with only 20% resolving spontaneously after an additional 3 months, 25% after 6 months, and 30% after 1 year [17].The guidelines specify that while the otolaryngologist should offer BMTT, the final decision should be based on discussion with the child's caregivers regarding the poor natural history of COME, the risks and benefits of BMTT, and that the main alternative to surgical intervention is further surveillance [1].

3. *BMTT may be performed in children with unilateral or bilateral OME of less than 3 months duration if they also have symptoms that are attributable to OME, such as balance issues, poor school performance, behavioral issues, ear discomfort, and reduced QOL* [1]. BMTT in this setting may reduce symptoms of MEE while eliminating the MEE as a confounding factor in work-up of vestibular complaints, otalgia, and social issues. OME has been shown to have a negative impact on the vestibular system, and these deficiencies may resolve promptly after BMTT [1]. Additionally, children with OME have been shown to have increased behavioral problems; attention disorders; mood disorders; and difficulties with speech, reading, and vocabulary [27, 28].

4. *Children with COME who do not receive BMTT should be re-evaluated at 3- to 6-month intervals until the effusion has resolved, significant HL is detected, or structural abnormalities of the TM or ME are suspected* [1]. MEE contains inflammatory mediators that can potentially induce structural changes of the TM [29, 30]. Negative pressure in the ME can also produce retraction pockets, atelectasis, or cholesteatoma over time. The longer the effusion is present, the higher the risk of structural damage. Thus, the ears in a child with OME should be monitored periodically for changes. Reassessment also allows for

detection of HL that may develop during surveillance. This is important as children with moderate HL of 40 dB or greater are at risk for problems with speech and language which may impair behavior [27, 31] and school performance [32].

5. *BMTT should not be performed in children with RAOM if they do not have MEE at the time of surgical assessment, unless the child is "at-risk"* (including those with antibiotic intolerance/allergy, complications of OM (mastoiditis, meningitis, facial nerve paralysis), developmental delay, immunosuppression, or severe/persistent AOM) [1]. RCTs looking at antibiotic prophylaxis for RAOM without OME showed that children taking a placebo had a reduction in episodes of RAOM from a baseline of 5.5 or more annually to 2.8 annual episodes [17]. This suggests the natural history of RAOM trends toward improvement. Several reviews have indicated that TTs had only a transient benefit for decreasing the incidence of RAOM [13, 26, 33]. Casselbrant et al. have demonstrated a modest decrease of 30 days per year in the time children had with MEE once tubes were placed [34]. Other studies have shown similar modest improvements but were performed with short-lasting (Paparella type I) tubes. Longer-lasting grommet-style tubes may be expected to provide a greater effusion-free period of time. A more recent RCT found significant benefits in prevention of RAOM after BMTT in children aged 10 months to 2 years; however, this study included children with OME at the time of surgery leading to the guideline recommendation for placing tubes only if MEE is present at the time of evaluation [35].

This aspect of the guideline is perhaps the most controversial as it may delay intervention for children who will eventually require TTs, children may continue to require systemic antibiotic therapy for AOM events, and there is a high tendency for relapse of OME even if the ear is clear during evaluation. This also may lead to confusion among caregivers and animosity between primary care providers and otolaryngologists regarding diagnosis and management of these children. Prior guidelines published by the American Academy of Pediatrics recommended offering BMTT for RAOM consisting of three episodes in 6 months or four episodes in 1 year with one episode in the preceding 6 months [19]. Specialists may find that many pediatricians still refer patients based on this guideline; therefore, the decision not to perform BMTT in children without OME may contradict the desires of pediatricians and frustrate caregivers. There is also additional evidence that TTs do decrease the risk of RAOM. A Danish analysis of five RCTs with a total of 519 children showed that BMTT prevented one episode of AOM for every 6 months they are in place. Additionally, they keep one of three otitis-prone children free of AOM in the first 6 months [36].

6. *BMTT should be offered to children with RAOM who have unilateral or bilateral OME at the time of assessment* [1]. This guideline is supported by multiple RCTs; however, the heterogeneity of the trials makes the magnitude of clinical benefit difficult to discern. Two RCTs including children with RAOM who had MEE showed a decrease in the average number of AOM episodes by 2.5 per child-year [37, 38]. In an RCT of children under age 2 years with MEE and RAOM, BMTT reduced subsequent episodes of AOM by 0.55 per child-year. This decrease, while modest, was significant [35]. Additional studies also showed children with OME of 2 months duration or greater who underwent BMTT had reduction of future episodes of AOM. Again, the improvement was modest at 0.20–0.72 fewer episodes per child-year [39]. Despite the variability in improvement, the studies confirm that there is a benefit to BMTT in children with RAOM and evidence of MEE.

7. Presence of MEE at the time of assessment may provide some reassurance that prior diagnoses of AOM were accurate, as well as support that Eustachian tube (ET) function is impaired. BMTT is recommended even if the MEE is unilateral as ET function is thought to be similar on both sides in more than 70 % of children [40]. BMTT carried an added benefit

during episodes of AOM while the tubes are patent allowing treatment with topical antibiotic drops, resulting in decreasing pain, less exposure to systemic antibiotics, and shorter periods of hearing impairment.

8. *BMTT may be performed in "at-risk" children with unilateral or bilateral OME that is unlikely to resolve quickly.* This includes children who have a flat, type B tympanogram or OME lasting 3 or more months [1]. As previously discussed, it is important to identify children who may be less tolerant of setbacks from AOM and OME. Children with preexisting SNHL could have substantial difficulty if a 20-dB CHL were to complicate the situation, worsening existing speech and language delays or negating the benefits of hearing aids [41, 42]. Children with visual disturbances, developmental and behavioral disorders, Down syndrome, cleft palate, and other craniofacial syndromes are specifically targeted in this statement. While there are no controlled trials supporting the beneficial impact of BMTT in "at-risk" children, the panel agreed that BMTT is a reasonable intervention for reducing prevalence of MEE that would otherwise have low likelihood of spontaneous resolution and may place those children at high risks for HL [1].

The guidelines are written based on the assumption that resolution of an MEE will improve speech and language function. The evidence on this topic is controversial with few studies looking at this endpoint in a truly representative population. A Cochrane Review by Browning examined ten trials involving more than 1700 children. The authors concluded that grommets had no effect on speech or language development, behavior, or cognitive function. There are, however, many flaws in this study and its conclusions. First, it largely includes a population of older, relatively asymptomatic children, so the study was not designed for seeing improvements in speech or language developments. As noted in Hoerr's law, "it is difficult to make an asymptomatic patient better" [43]. While OM is mainly a disease of young children, those under the age of 3 were excluded in this review, as

were children with disabilities or other medical comorbidities, making the results less applicable. The authors did note an improvement in hearing of 10 dB with BMTT, but this was felt to be trivial. In "at-risk" children, however, the effects of this hearing improvement may be more significant [24, 44]. The authors concluded that benefits of grommets were short lived, lasting only for the 6–9 months while the Paparella type I tubes were in place [24]. A longer-lasting short-term tube may have shown a longer duration of benefit. Finally, the authors focused only on the outcome of HL, ignoring other important aspects of the disease, such as subsequent infections with need for further antibiotics, fever, pain, impaired sleep, QOL, and parent satisfaction [24]. Similar issues were seen in a study by Paradise consisting of 429 healthy children under the age of 3 with persistent MEE randomized to undergo BMTT or wait 9 months to undergo BMTT if the effusion remained. Between the ages 9 and 11, 391 of those same children were assessed for literacy, attention, social skills, and academic achievement. The authors found no significant differences in 48 developmental measures between children who underwent early or delayed BMTT [45]. The indications for TT placement at that time, however, were much more lax than the current ones as they did not take into account hearing thresholds, speech or language delay, or other comorbidities. Additionally, only 27% of the children had bilateral effusions lasting longer than 90 days, and children now considered "at-risk" were excluded. Less than half of the children would meet current surgical criteria, and 60% had only unilateral effusions, which would not be expected to interfere with developmental outcomes. A more appropriate conclusion may have been that there is no long-term benefit to early BMTT in otherwise healthy, normal children with minor HL and no preexisting speech or language issues.

Other studies addressing developmental outcomes suggested mild negative effects of OM; however, a relatively healthy population of children without significant risk factors again limits the application of these results. A meta-analysis of 11 studies by Roberts revealed children with a history of OM had poorer receptive and expressive language at age 2–5 years than those without a history of OM ($p<0.01$), as did those with worse hearing at ages 1–2 years ($p<0.01$). The authors could not associate receptive or expressive speech milestones with OME and HL and felt these had only a very small negative effect on future speech and language development in otherwise healthy children [46]. Golz performed a case-control study of 80 otitis-prone children, with a history of greater than ten episodes of AOM by age 5 years and a speech reception threshold (SRT) over 25 dB. They were compared to 80 otitis-free children at ages 6.5–8 years for reading outcomes. The otitis-prone group had a higher mean number of reading mistakes at 15 versus 6% in the otitis-free group ($p<0.001$). They concluded that a history of RAOM with HL before the age of 5 may put children at an educational disadvantage interfering with reading skills [47]. While OM is a common feature of childhood for many children, in the presence of comorbidities, HL, or speech/language difficulties, early intervention may mediate these negative effects on developmental outcomes.

It is important to note that the guidelines strongly emphasize shared decision-making with the child's caregiver when choosing a course of treatment. The physician should discuss with caregivers the potential risks and benefits of the surgery, as well as what to expect once the TTs are in place. Particularly, the expected amount of the time the TTs will stay in place, the follow-up needs, and how complications are detected should be pointed out [1]. Unfortunately, the guidelines did not provide any insight into which types of TT to use in various situations, the role of adenoidectomy or control of allergies, indications for repeat TT placement, whether to use drops after tube insertion, how to deal with a plugged tube, indications for removal of TTs, or the nuances of water precautions.

Tympanostomy Tube Types

Wide arrays of TT options are available varying in shape, size, and materials. The ideal TT would be easy to insert with a predictable time to extru-

sion; improve RAOM, COME, and hearing; and not have complications [48]. Surprisingly, there are few studies that assess the efficacy of certain types of tubes over others in achieving these goals.

A major distinction between tubes is if they are short term or long term. Short-term tubes typically last anywhere from 6 to 24 months and are indicated for most children who undergo initial TT placement. Armstrong and Shepard grommets are the most common short-term TTs used by otolaryngologists in the USA [12, 49], with mean times to tube extrusions of approximately 16.5 months and 8.5 months, respectively [48, 50]. The mean times to extrusion for Paparella type I tubes and Reuter Bobbin tubes, both short-acting, are 7 months and 17 months, respectively [51]. Long-term tubes, on the other hand, are generally reserved for children, adolescents, and adults who have required multiple sets of TTs due to failure of resolution of disease after short-acting TT placement. Modified Goode T-tubes, butterfly, Triune, and Paparella II are the most commonly used long-acting TT designs. These tubes can last from several months to years [52].

Tube positioning in the TM has been studied in relation to its effect on duration of action. Placement in the anterior-superior quadrant was thought to portend up to fourfold increased time till extrusion versus placement in either the anterior- or posterior-inferior quadrants in an early study [53]. More recent investigations, however, have shown no difference in the time to extrusion between tubes placed in the anterior-inferior and anterior-superior quadrants [54−56]. Placement in the posterior quadrant was associated with significantly earlier tube extrusion in two thirds of 52 patients in one study. This finding was thought to be due to keratin migration patterns of the squamous layer of the TM [57]. The most important factors affecting duration of tube retention seem to be principally related to the tube properties, including the length, diameter, and flanges of the tube [52]. For example, Paparella II tubes have a wider inner diameter of 1.42 mm versus around 1.1 mm for most short-term tubes. Modified Goode T-tubes have inner flanges at least 5 mm longer than short-acting tubes, as well as no outer flanges. Longer inner flanges or lack of outer flanges make it more difficult for the keratin accumulating on the surface of the TM to push the TT out [57].

Other nuances that may affect TT choice include material type and the presence of beveling or flanges. Various tube materials are available, including polyethylene, silastic (Silicone), fluoroplastic (Teflon), and titanium. These are all relatively inert materials, but there are subtle differences between the tubes that have been studied in effort to determine the ideal tube. Metal tubes have a smoother surface, which has potential for being more bacteria-resistant [58]. However, 31 children had more granulation tissue in ears with titanium tubes and a nonsignificant trend toward increased otorrhea rates as compared with Shepard fluoroplastic tubes. The titanium tubes were also more likely to prematurely extrude with 43 % coming out within 12 months postoperatively versus only 7 % of the fluoroplastic tubes [59]. Another study of 86 children with fluoroplastic tubes in one ear and silicone tubes in the other showed less otorrhea in the first 3 weeks postoperatively with fluoroplastic tubes [60]. In a prospective, randomized study in which children had Goode T-tubes placed in one ear and one of three short-term tubes (Shepard fluoroplastic, Reuter Bobbin, or Armstrong beveled) in the other, several differences were noted. T-tubes, had longer rates of retention. There was no difference in mean times to extrusion among the three short-term tubes. T-tubes, as expected, had increased rates of otorrhea, while Shepard fluoroplastic had significantly lower rates of otorrhea. The rates of otorrhea were intermediate for both Reuter Bobbin and Armstrong beveled tubes. The Reuter Bobbin tubes, with an inner diameter of only 1.0 mm, had the highest rate of obstruction [51]. Other studies suggest that tube obstruction rate is solely a function of the tube diameter as there were no differences between TT types of the same diameter [58, 61]. The most commonly used materials by US surgeons are fluoroplastic and silastic [49]. Various antibiotic or anti-inflammatory drug-eluting TTs as well as silver oxide coated TTs have been developed in efforts to reduce post-TT otorrhea by reducing biofilm formation and development of resistant bacteria. Unfortunately, none have proven to be terribly efficacious up to this point.

Tube selection should be individualized to the patient. Children with craniofacial syndromes and suspected long-term ET dysfunction should be considered for long-term TTs sooner than otherwise healthy children. Similarly, children with small ear canals may require special consideration. Specifically, young children with Down syndrome often require small-diameter tubes (Tiny Tef, Mini-Shah, Mini-Shay) as larger tubes will not fit through the external auditory canal (EAC) [52]. As the diameter is smaller, these tubes are more prone to earlier extrusion and occlusion. Silicone tubes, which are more flexible, may be another option for children with small canals; however, they are more difficult to place due to their pliability. Also, severe atelectasis may obliterate the ME space in some children making it difficult to place a tube with large inner flanges. Surgeons should be comfortable placing a variety of TTs depending on what is most appropriate for the child's specific situation.

Role of Adenoidectomy

The role of adenoidectomy in management of OM is complex. Enlarged adenoids may prevent resolution of MEE by physical obstruction of the ET orifice in the nasopharynx. The adenoids have long been thought to serve as a reservoir for pathogens that can cause inflammation, thus disrupting ET function. Biofilms were shown to be more prevalent in children with adenoid hypertrophy and COME than in those with adenoid hypertrophy alone (74 vs. 42 %), as was bacteria presence in adenoid tissue by polymerase chain reaction (PCR; 96 vs. 48 %) [62]. Many otolaryngologists choose to perform adenoidectomy in children who require a second set of TTs or those with severe ME disease in conjunction with signs and symptoms of nasal obstruction, sleep apnea, or recurrent adenoiditis. While the recently published guidelines did not make recommendations on this topic, multiple studies have addressed the issue.

A retrospective case review of more than 2100 consecutive children who underwent BMTT at a tertiary children's hospital over a 5-year period looked at risk factors for requiring more than one set of TTs. Of that group, nearly 20 % required a second set of tubes within 3 years of initial surgery. Children under the age of 18 months at the time of the initial surgery were almost twice as likely to require replacement of the tubes after extrusion ($p < 0.005$). If the child had an adenoidectomy in conjunction with the first or second BMTT, however, it reduced the need for an additional set of TTs by a factor of 3 ($p < 0.001$). If adenoidectomy was not performed with the second BMTT, children had a 40 % risk of requiring additional sets of TTs. Other risk factors identified for needing more than one set of TTs were craniofacial deformity and family history of ear, nose, and throat (ENT)-related surgery [63]. A more recent retrospective review of 904 children treated at an academic hospital over a 7-year period also showed very similar findings. Of children who underwent BMTT without adenoidectomy, 20 % required an additional set of tubes versus only 7 % in children who had adenoidectomy with initial BMTT ($p < 0.0001$). This study showed that children between the ages 4 and 10 years had the most benefit from adenoidectomy in terms of preventing repeat tube insertion ($p < 0.0001$) [64]. The largest study on the topic is a retrospective review of outcomes in more than 50,000 children during a 24-year period in Australia. In this study, children undergoing BMTT alone were compared with those who had an adenoidectomy and/or tonsillectomy performed in addition to the BMTT. The risk of requiring additional BMTT was reduced by 16, 17, and 10 % in children having adenoidectomy alone, tonsillectomy alone, or tonsillectomy and adenoidectomy, respectively ($p < 0.001$). If adenoidectomy or tonsillectomy and adenoidectomy were performed with the second set of TTs, the risk of a having a third set was reduced by 15 and 17 %, respectively ($p < 0.001$); however, there was no difference with tonsillectomy alone [65]. In an RCT from Finland, younger children with RAOM were studied to assess the benefits of early adenoidectomy. The study con-

sisted of 300 children aged 10 months to 2 years with RAOM who were randomized to undergo BMTT alone, BMTT with adenoidectomy, or no surgical intervention. The control group had a 34 % failure rate, which was significantly higher than the BMTT alone group (21 %, $p = 0.04$) and the BMTT with adenoidectomy group (16 %, $p = 0.004$). The authors concluded that in children under the age of 2 years, BMTT was effective at preventing RAOM with or without adenoidectomy [35].

While adenoidectomy appears beneficial in reducing the risk of developing additional ME disease that would require surgery, there are obvious risks to including adenoidectomy along with placement of TTs. These include the need for endotracheal intubation and administration of intravenous anesthetics, and the possibility of bleeding, infection, and velopharyngeal insufficiency. It is our stance that children who require placement of a second set of tubes (or those who have symptoms of nasal obstruction or recurrent rhinorrhea at the time of their initial tube placement) should be considered for an examination of the adenoids under anesthesia with removal if enlarged or obstructive [63]. Further studies are needed to determine which children may benefit the most from adenoidectomy as some believe that the procedure is beneficial regardless of their size.

Complications

TT placement for OM has multiple benefits including improving hearing by 5–12 dB [25], decreasing effusion prevalence by 32 % [12], and reduction in the incidence of RAOM. The procedure can also provide improved QOL as well as a mechanism for drainage and for the administration of topical antibiotic therapy. They may also reduce suppurative complications, damage to the TM, adverse effects of antibiotics, and potential developmental sequelae of HL [61]. However, as with any surgical procedure, there are risks involved. The risk of general anesthesia cannot be overlooked. The incidence of anesthesia-related death for children undergoing surgery ranges from 1/10,000 to 1/45,000. Children are more prone to laryngospasm and bronchospasm, thus increasing risk of anesthetic complications [66]. A prospective review of 1000 children who underwent BMTT at a tertiary children's hospital showed that only 9% of patients experienced a minor adverse event (upper airway obstruction, prolonged recovery, emesis, post-procedural agitation), mostly attributable to agitation or prolonged recovery. Moreover, major complications (cardiopulmonary events like laryngospasm, stridor, or dysrhythmia) occurred only in 1.9% of children. Children with acute or chronic illness were 2.78 times more likely to develop an adverse event ($p < 0.001$). Importantly, no admissions, required consultations of other services, or deaths were noted during the study [67].

Sequelae of TTs themselves are common but transient (i.e., otorrhea) or do not generally affect function (i.e., tympanosclerosis, focal atrophy, shallow retraction pocket). Sometimes, tubes extrude too soon or get occluded, making them nonfunctional. The most problematic, but thankfully rahter rare, complications are residual TM perforations and cholesteatoma.

Short-Term Complications

A meta-analysis aiming to estimate complications related to TT placement reviewed 134 articles. The most common complication was transient otorrhea, occurring in 17% of patients. In the early postoperative period, 16% of children developed otorrhea, whereas 26% developed otorrhea at any point while the TT remained in place. Recurrent or chronic otorrhea were rare, seen in only 7.4 and 3.8% of children, respectively. Otorrhea is 2.2 times more likely with long-term TTs [61].

The recently published guidelines recommend prescribing topical antibiotic eardrops, without oral antibiotics, for children with uncomplicated otorrhea [1]. Ototopical drops approved for use with TTs include ciprofloxacin-dexamethasone (Ciprodex) and ofloxacin. These drops are highly efficacious in treating suppurative otorrhea caused by the most common AOM pathogens, as well as *Pseudomonas aeruginosa* and *Staphylo-*

coccus aureus. This method avoids the unnecessary delivery of systemic antibiotics and their potential side effects. The drugs are also delivered in higher concentration to the site of infection, thus potentially reducing the risk of drug-resistance. Topical antibiotic and/or steroid eardrop placement intraoperatively may help prevent blockage of TTs and early postoperative otorrhea, but the evidence is controversial. In a meta-analysis of nine studies, only three showed a statistically significant benefit to prophylactic drop placement. However, all nine studies showed a trend toward benefit of drops, and the collective result showed significant decrease in otorrhea with drop placement with an odds ratio (OR) of 0.52 [68]. An RCT compared a control group with no prophylaxis, a group receiving gentamicin otic drops in the OR only, and a third group that received gentamicin drops after surgery for a total of 48 h. Postoperative otorrhea rates were 12, 8.8, and 5.6%, respectively, which, despite a trend toward benefit with prophylaxis, did not reach statistical significance ($p = 0.62$). There was, on the other hand, a highly significant benefit of the use of drops when a mucoid or purulent MEE was noted at the time of surgery ($p < 0.001$) [67]. Regardless of the potential reduction in otorrhea, the risk of ototoxicity with certain drops, such as neomycin-polymixin B or gentamicin, must be taken into account. Ofloxacin drops may provide the benefit of decreased otorrhea with a favorable side-effect profile.

Other common complications seen with TTs in the short term included occlusion of the tube lumen in 7%, granulation tissue in 4%, premature extrusion in 3.9%, and displacement into the ME in 0.5% of ears. Granulation tissue development required removal of the TT or debridement in the operating room in 1.8% of cases [61]. Intrusion into the ME, though rare, may require ME exploration for removal.

While not necessarily a complication, water precautions are an issue that must be addressed with TT placement. Historically, parents had been instructed to have their children avoid water exposure in the presence of ventilation tubes, either by avoiding swimming or protecting the ears during swimming and bathing. This was based on the premise that water will pass through the

TT and enter the ME space, thus introducing bacteria to the ME and causing infection. However, theoretical models have shown that water passage into the ME does not occur as easily as one might think [67–69]. Additionally, multiple studies have shown no benefit in reducing otorrhea with water avoidance, use of ear protection (i.e., earplugs, bathing caps), or prophylactic eardrops in most cases. Salata and Derkay conducted a prospective trial enrolling 533 patients divided into four groups of swimming without water precautions, using antibiotic eardrops after swimming, using earplugs with swimming, and non-swimming. The rates of swimming-related otorrhea were 11, 14, and 20% in the swimming groups. The overall rates of otorrhea were 59% in the non-swimming group and 68% in the swimming groups combined ($p=0.11$) [70] A randomized study on the topic examined 200 children randomized to either swimming with or without earplugs and noted no significant difference in the rates of otorrhea at 47 and 56%, respectively. However, there was a significant difference in the number of episodes of otorrhea per month at 0.07 with earplugs and 0.10 without earplugs ($p=0.05$). The clinical importance of this, on the other hand, correlates to only 0.36 infections per child per year and would require a child to wear earplugs for 2.8 years to prevent one infection [71].

Children with TT appear to be at minimal, if any, risk for increased otorrhea with water exposure when surface swimming in pools or ocean water [72]. Exposure to soapy water or river/lake water is controversial. The decreased surface tension and increased bacterial counts may increase the risk of water entering the ME and infection, respectively [69, 73]. Restrictions after TT placement could prevent acquisition of life-saving water skills and impose unnecessary expense and difficulty on families. Both a recent review of the literature and the guidelines agree that clinicians should not routinely recommend water precautions after TT placement [1, 72]. While not addressed by the guidelines, jumping and diving are probably best avoided as the risk of water entering the ME increases with swimming at greater depths [73, 74].

Long-Term Complications

Long-term complications include TM changes, HL, perforations of the TM, and cholesteatoma. Myringosclerosis consists of white patches in the TM caused by calcium deposits. It is seen more commonly in ears that have previously had TTs, occurring in approximately 32% of ears after tube extrusion, than in those who have not [61]. It is usually limited to the TM and does not cause appreciable HL [12, 26, 61]. HL of 1–2 dB was shown in children after TT as compared with those who did not have TTs. Hearing was usually still within normal range and the loss was not clinically significant [75]. Atrophy of the TM, atelectasis, and retraction pockets are also more common in children with OM who have been treated with TTs [76]. The former two findings were seen in about 25% of ears after TTs, but retraction pockets were observed in only 3.1%. Short- versus long-term tube presence did not affect the incidence of tube obstruction, myringosclerosis, atrophy, or retraction pockets [61].

More troublesome complications occur most often when failure of tube extrusion occurs. Beyond 30 months postoperatively, TTs are unlikely to extrude spontaneously [77]. Rates of TTs retention vary with different tube types and may necessitate a return trip to the operating room for removal. Patch repair of the perforation at time of tube removal has shown mixed results with regard to healing of perforation as compared with no patch [78–80]. Perforation is more likely to occur if TTs are retained beyond 36 months (40%) versus those that are in less than 36 months (19%) [78]. Chronic TM perforation was noted in 4.8% of more than 20,000 ears from a combined 62 studies. The incidence for short-term TTs was 2.2 versus 16.6% in long-term TTs. Similarly, rates of cholesteatoma development were higher in patients with long-term TTs (1.4%) versus short-term ones (0.8%). The overall rate of cholesteatoma was 0.7% in nearly 15,000 ears from 33 studies examined [61].

Emerging Technologies

The placement of TTs is a well-established procedure; however, new technologies are being developed in hopes of improving ease of surgery, underlying causes of disease, and patient outcomes. The Acclarent Tympanostomy Tube Delivery System, which allows for automated TT deployment, is one of these developments. The system was prospectively tested in 53 patients under the age of 5 years. Deployment was successful in 94 % of attempts and the tubes remained in place and patent 1 week postoperatively in 99 % of patients. This advancement may allow for future in-office placement of TTs when combined with improved ionophoresis systems [81]. With the changing environment of high-deductible in healthcare, more parents may seek care performed in a doctor's office under local anesthesia when possible.

Other investigators have looked at making the tube itself more effective. A biodegradable drug-eluting tube has been tested to potentially treat patients suffering from COME. Collar button tubes were loaded with the antibiotic, ofloxacin, and designed to slowly elute the drug over a 3-month period. When tested in guinea pigs, the tubes resulted in no inflammation or episodes of otorrhea. The drug-eluting tubes had the least bacteria adherence when compared with Mini Shah TTs and biodegradable TTs without the drug. The tubes began degrading by 18 weeks after placement and had eluded approximately 82 % of the drug by the 3-month mark. These tubes have the potential for reducing biofilm development and the benefit of not having retained tubes requiring removal [82]. Another method of improving management of patients with OME is balloon dilation of the ET. Eleven patients, all with a long-standing history of COME and multiple sets of TTs, underwent dilation of the cartilaginous portion of the ET using sinus dilation balloons inflated up to 12 atm pressure for 1 min via an endoscopic transnasal approach while under general anesthesia. At up to 14 months follow-up, the subjects, all of whom were previously unable to autoinsufflate their ET, were found to be able to

self-insufflate using a Valsalva maneuver after the procedure. Moreover, the atelectasis in the ears resolved in all cases, and no complications were noted [83]. It is hoped that this technology will be able to be applied to children with chronic Eustachian tube dysfunction (ETD) in the future.

Conclusions

TT placement is a very common procedure performed in the pediatric population. Indications for surgery include OME or RAOM meeting evidence-based requirements. Families of patients should be involved in making decisions about whether or not to perform surgery. If surgery is performed, various types of tubes are available. Long-term tubes are associated with a higher incidence of otorrhea, perforation, and cholesteatoma although they are typically only placed in children with more significant or recalcitrant ETD. The majority of complications associated with TT placement, however, are transient or not clinically significant. The decision to place TTs and their care thereafter should be individualized based on the patient and the overall clinical picture.

References

1. Rosenfeld RM, Schwartz SR, Pynnonen MA, Tunkel DE, Hussey HM, Fichera JS, Grimes AM, Hackell JM, Farrison MF, Haskell H, Haynes DS, Kim TW, Lafrenierre DC, Netterville JL, Pipan ME, Raol NP, Schellhase KG. Clinical practice guidelines: tympanostomy tubes in children. Otolaryngology Head Neck Surg. 2013;149(s 1):1–35.
2. Bluestone CD, Swarts JD. Human evolutionary history: Consequences for the pathogenesis of otitis media. Otolaryngology Head Neck Surg. 2004;130(suppl 5):S95–118.
3. Casselbrant ML, Mandel EM. Epidemiology. In: Rosenfeld RM, Bluestone DC, editors. Evidence-based otitis media. 2 nd edn. Hamilton: BC Decker; 2003. p. 147–62. Print.
4. Daly KA, Hoffman HJ, Kvaerner KJ, et al. Epidemiology, natural history, and risk factors: panel report from the ninth international research conference on otitis media. Int J Pediatr Otorhinolaryngol. 2010;74:231–40.

5. Casselbrant ML, Mandel EM. Acute otitis media and otitis media with effusion. In: Paul WF, Bruce HH, Valerie JL, John NN, Mark AR, editors. Cummings otolaryngology—head and neck surgery. 5 th edn. Philadelphia: Mosby Elseiver; 2010. p. 2761–77. Print.

6. Wallace IF, Berkman ND, Lohr KN, Harrison MF, Kimple AJ, Steiner MJ. Surgical treatments for otitis media with effusion: a systematic review. Pediatrics. 2014;133:296–311.

7. Freid VM, Makuc DM, Rooks RN. Ambulatory health care visits by children: principal diagnosis and place of visit. Vital Health Stat 13. 1998;137:1–23.

8. Woodwell DA. Office visits to otolaryngologists 1989–90, National Ambulatory Medical Care Survey. Adv Data. 1992;222:1–11.

9. Barber C, Ille S, Vergisonc A, Coates H. Acute otitis media in young children—What do parents say? Int J Pediatr Otorhinolaryngol. 2014;78(2):300–6.

10. Maron T, Tan A, Wilkinson GS, Pierson KS, Freeman JL, Chonmaitree T. Trends in otitis media-related health care use in the United States, 2001–2011. JAMA Pediatrics. 2014;168(1):68–75.

11. Centers for Disease Control and Prevention. Table 2: top 5 diagnoses at visits to office-based physicians and hospital outpatient departments by patient age and sex: United States 2008. In: National Ambulatory Health Care Survey 2008. Atlanta: Centers for Disease Control and Prevention; 2008.

12. Browning GG, Rovers MM, Williamson I, Lous J, Burton MJ. Grommets (ventilation tubes) for hearing loss associated with otitis media with effusion in children. Cochrane Database Syst Rev. 2010;10:CD001801.

13. Rosenfeld RM, Bhaya MH, Bower CM, et al. Impact of tympanostomy tubes on child quality of life. Arch Otolaryngol Head Neck Surg. 2000;126(5):585–92.

14. Cullen KA, Hall MJ, Golosinskiy A. Ambulatory surgery in the United States, 2006. National Health Stat Rep. 2009;11:1–25.

15. Wolleswinkel-van den Bosch JH, Stolk EA, Francoi M, Gasparini R, Brosa M. The heath care burden and societal impact of acute otitis media in seven European countries: results of an Internet survey. Vaccine. 2010;28(suppl 6):G39–52.

16. Teele DW, Klein JO, Rosner BA. Epidemiology of otitis media in children. Ann Otol Rhinol Laryngol Suppl. 1980;89(3 pt 2):5–6.

17. Rosenfeld RM, Kay DJ. Natural history of untreated otitis media. Laryngoscope. 2003;113(10):1645–57.

18. Williamson IG, Dunleavey J, Bain J, Robinson D. The natural history of otitis media with effusion—a three-year study of the incidence and prevalence of abnormal tympanograms in four South West Hampshire infant and first schools. J Laryngol Otol. 1994;108(11):930–4.

19. Lieberthal AS, Carroll AE, Chonmaitree T, Ganiats TG, Hoberman A, Jackson MA, Joffe MD, Miller DT, Rosenfeld RM, Sevilla XD, Schwartz RH, Thomas PA, Tunkel DE. The diagnosis and management of acute otitis media. Pediatrics. 2013;131:e964.

20. Lambert E, Roy S. Otitis media and ear tubes. Pediatr Clin North Am. 2013;60(4):809–26.

21. Gravel JS. Hearing and auditory function. In: Rosenfeld RM, Bluestone CD, editors. Evidence-based otitis media. 2 nd edition. Hamilton: BC Decker; 2003. p. 342–59.

22. Fria TJ, Cantekin EI, EIchler JA. Hearing acuity of children with otitis media with effusion. Arch Otolaryngol. 1985;111(1):10–6.

23. Rosenfeld RM, Jang D, Tarashansky K. Tympanostomy tube outcomes in children at-risk and not-at-risk for developmental delays. Int J Pediatr Otorhinolaryngol. 2011;75:190–5.

24. Burton MJ, Derkay CS, Rosenfeld RM. Extracts from *The Cochrane Library* Grommets (Ventilation Tubes) for hearing loss associated with otitis media with effusion in children. Otolaryngol Head Neck Surg. 2011;144(5):657–61.

25. Rovers MM, Black N, Browning GG, Maw R, Zielhuis GA, Haggard MP. Grommets in otitis media with effusion: an individual patient data meta-analysis. Arch Dis Child. 2005;90(5):480–5.

26. Hellstrom S, Groth A, Jorgensen F, et al. Ventilation tube treatment: a systematic review of the literature. Otolaryngol Head Neck Surg. 2011;145(3):383–95.

27. Haggard MP, Birkin JA, Browning GG, Gatehouse S, Lewis S. Behavior problems in otitis media. Pediatr Infect Dis J. 1994;13(1 suppl 1):S43–50.

28. Gouma P, Mallis A, Daniilidis V, Gouveris H, Armenakis N, Maxakis S. Behavioral trends in young children with conductive hearing loss: a case-control study. Eur Arch Otorhinolaryngol. 2011;268(1):63–6.

29. Piche Yellon RF, Doyle WJ, Whiteside TL, Diven WF, March AR, Fireman P. Cytokines, immunoglobulins, and bacterial pathogens in middle ear effusion. Arch Otolaryngol Head Neck Surg. 1995;121(8):865–9 Pichichero ME. Aucte otitis media: Part I. Improving diagnostic accuracy. Am Fam Physician. 2000;61(7):2051–6.

30. Samuel EA, Burrows A, Kerschner JE. Cytokine regulation of mucin secretion in a human middle ear epithelial model. Cytokine. 2008;41(1):38–43.

31. Mitchell RB, Kelly J. Child behavior after adenotonsillectomy for obstructive sleep apnea syndrome. Laryngoscope. 2005;115:2051–5.

32. Rosenfeld RM, Culpepper L, Doyle KJ, et al. Clinical practice guideline: otitis media with effusion. Otolaryngol Head Neck Surg. 2004;130(suppl 5):S95–118.

33. McDonald S, Langton Hewer CD, Nunez DA. Grommets (ventilation tubes) for recurrent acute otitis media in children. Cochrane Database Syst Rev. 2008;(4):CD004741.

34. Casselbrant ML, Kaleida PH, Rockette HE, et al. Efficacy of antimicrobial prophylaxis and of tympanostomy tube insertion for prevention of recurrent acute otitis media: results of a randomized clinical trial. Pediatr Infect Dis J. 1992;11(4):278–86.

35. Kujala T, Alho OP, Luotonen J, Krista A, Uhari M, Renko M, Kontiokari T, Pokka T, Koivunen P. Tympanstomy with and without adenoidectomy for the prevention of recurrences of acute otitis media: a randomized controlled trial. Pediatr Infect Dis J. 2012;31(6):565–9.

36. Lous J, Ryborg CT, Thomsen JL. A systematic review of the effect of tympanostomy tubes in children with recurrent acute otitis media. Int J Pediatr Otorhinolaryngol. 2011;75:1058–61.

37. Gebhart DE. Tympanostomy tubes in the otitis media prone child. Laryngoscope. 1981;91(6):849–66.

38. Gonzalez C, Arnold JE, Woody EA, et al. Prevention of recurrent acute otitis media: chemoprophylaxis versus tympanostomy tubes. Laryngoscope. 1978;88(7 pt 1):1139–54.

39. Mandel EM, Rockette HE, Bluestone DC, Paradise JL, Nozza RJ. Efficacy of myringotomy with and without tympanostomy tubes for chronic otitis media with effusion. Pediatr Infect Dis J. 1992;115(10):1217–24.

40. van Heerbeek N, Akkerman AE, Ingels KJAO, Entel JAM, Zielhuis GA. Left-right differences in Eustachian tube function in children with ventilation tubes. Int J Pediatr Otorhinolaryngol. 2003;67:861–6.

41. Ruben RJ, Math R. Serous otitis media associated with a sensorineural hearing loss in children. Laryngoscope. 1978;88(7 pt 1):1139–54.

42. Brookhouser PE, Worthington DW, Kelly WJ. Middle ear disease in young children with sensorineural hearing loss. Laryngoscope. 1993;103(4 pt 1):371–8.

43. Hoerr SO. Hoerr's law. Am J Surg. 1962;103:411.

44. Rosenfeld RM, Jang D, Tarashansky K. Tympanostomy tube outcomes in children at-risk and not-at-risk for developmental delays. Int J Pediatr Otorhinolaryngol. 2011;75:190–5.

45. Paradise JL, Feldman HM, Campbell TF, Gollaghan CA, Rockette HE, Pitcairn DL, Smith CG, Colborn DK, Bernard BS, Kurs-Lasky M, Janosky JE, Sabo DL, O'Connor RE, Pelham WE. Tympanostomy tubes and developmental outcomes at 9 to 11 years of age. NEJM. 2007;356:248–61.

46. Roberts JE, Rosenfeld RM, Zeisel SA. Otitis media and speech and language: a meta-analysis of prospective studies. Pediatrics. 2004;113:e238–48.

47. Golz A, Netzer A, Westerman ST, Wsterman LM, Gilbert DA, Joachims HZ, Golenberg D. Reading performance in children with otitis media. Otolaryngol Head Neck Surg. 2005;132:495–9.

48. Lindstrom DR, Reuben B, Jacobson K, Flanary VA, Kerschner JE. Long-term results of Armstrong beveled grommet tympanostomy tubes in children. Laryngoscope. 2004;114(3):490–4.

49. Todd WN. What your colleagues think of tympanostomy tubes—28 years later. Laryngoscope. 1999;109:1028–32.

50. Yaman H, Yilmaz S, Alkan N, Subasi B, Guclu E, Ozturk O. Shepard grommet tympanostomy tube complications in children with chronic otitis media with effusion. Eur Arch Otorhinolaryngol. 2010;267:1221–4.

51. Weigel MT, Parker MY, Manning M, et al. A prospective randomized study of four commonly used tympanostomy tubes. Laryngoscope. 1989;99:252–6.

52. Kay DJ. Type of tube to insert. In: Apler C, Bluestone C, Casselbrant M, Dohar J, Mandel E, editors. Advanced therapy of Otitis media. 1 st edition. Hamilton: BC Decker; 2004. p. 231–7. Print.

53. Armstrong BW. Prolonged middle ear ventilation: the right tube in the right place. Ann Otol Rhinol Laryngol. 1983;92(6 Pt 1):582–6.

54. April MM, Portella RR, Orobello PW Jr, Naclerio RM. Tympanostomy tube insertion: anterosuperior vs. anteroinferior quadrant. Otolaryngol Head Neck Surg. 1992;106(3):241–2.

55. Walker P. Ventilation tube duration versus site of placement. Aust N Z J Surg. 1997;67(8):571–2.

56. Hern JD, Jonathan DA. Insertion of ventilation tubes: does the site matter? Clin Otolaryngol Allied Sci. 1999;24(5):424–5.

57. van Baarle PW, Wentges RT. Extrusion of transtympanic ventilating tubes, relative to the site of insertion. ORL J Otorhinolaryngol Relat Spec. 1975;37(1):35–40.

58. Tami TA, Kennedy KS, Harley E. A clinical evaluation of gold-plated tubes for middle-ear ventilation. Arch Otolaryngol Head Neck Surg. 1987;113(9):979–80.

59. Shone GR, Griffith IP. Titanium grommets: a trial to assess function and extrusion rates. J Laryngol Otol. 1990;104(3):197–9.

60. Karlan MS, Skobel B, Grizzard M, Cassisi NJ, Singleton GT, Buscemi P, Goldberg EP. Myringotomy tube materials: bacterial adhesion and infection. Otolaryngol Head Neck Surg. 1980;88(6):783–94.

61. Kay DJ, Nelson M, Rosenfeld RM. Meta-analysis of tympanostomy tube sequelae. Otolaryngol Head Neck Surg. 2001;124:374–80

62. Safaan ME, Ibrahim WS, Tomoum MO. Role of adenoid biofilm in chronic otitis media with effusion in children. Eur Arch Otorhinolaryngol. 2013;270:2417–25.

63. Boston M, McCook J, Burke B, Derkay C. Incidence of and risk factors for additional tympanostomy tube insertion in children. Arch Otolaryngol Head Neck Surg. 2003;129:293–6.

64. Gleinser DM, Kriel KH, Mukerji S. The relationship between repeat tympanostomy tube insertion and adenoidectomy. Int J Pediatr Otorhinolaryngol. 2011;75:1247–51.

65. Kadhim AL, Spilsbury K, Semmens JB, Coates HL, Lannigan FJ. Adenoidectomy for middle ear effusion: a study of 50,000 children over 24 years. Laryngoscope. 2007;117:427–33.

66. van der Griend BF, Lister NA, McKenzie IM, et al. Postoperative mortality in children after 101,885 anesthetics at a tertiary pediatric hospital. Anesth Analg. 2011;112(6):1440–7.

67. Hoffman KK, Thompson GK, Burke BL, Derkay CS. Anesthetic complications of tympanostomy tube

placement in children. Arch Otolaryng Head Neck Surg. 2002;128:1040–3.

68. Scott BA, Strunk CL Jr. Post-tympanostomy otorrhea: a randomized clinical trial of topical prophylaxis. Otolaryng Head Neck Surg. 1992;106(1):34–41.

69. Marks NJ, Mills RP. Swimming and grommets. J R Soc Med. 1983; 76:23–6.

70. Wilcox LJ, Darrow DH. Should water precautions be recommended for children with tympanostomy tubes? Laryngoscope. 2014;124:10–11.

71. Salata JA, Derkay CS. Water precautions in children with tympanostomy tubes. Arch Otolaryngol. 1996;122:276–80.

72. Goldstein NA, Mandel EM, Kurs-Lasky M, Rockette HE, Casselbrant ML. Water precautions and tympanostomy tubes: a randomized, controlled trial. Laryngoscope. 2005;115:324–30.

73. Herbert RL, King GE, Bent JP. Tympanostomy tubes and water exposure: a practical model. Arch Otolaryngol. 1998;124:1118–21.

74. Lounsbury BF. Swimming unprotected with long-shafted middle ear ventilation tubes. Laryngoscope. 1985;95:340–3.

75. Johnston LC, Feldman HM, Paradise JL, et al. Tympanic membrane abnormalities and hearing levels at the ages of 4 and 5 years in relation to persistent otitis media and tympanostomy tube insertion in the first 3 years of life: a prospective study incorporating a randomized clinical trial. Pediatrics. 2004;114(1): e58–67.

76. De Beer BA, Schilder AG, Zielhuis GA, Graamans K. Natural course of tympanic membrane pathology related to totits media and ventilation tubes between ages 8 and 18 years. Otol Neurotol. 2005;26(5):1016–21.

77. Morris MS. Tympanostomy tubes: types, indications, techniques and complications. Otolaryngol Clin North Am. 1999;32:385–90.

78. Nichols PT, Ramadan HH, Wax MK, Santrock RD. Relationship between tympanic membrane perforations and retained ventilation tubes. Arch Otolaryngol Head Neck Surg. 1998;124:417–9.

79. El-Bitar MA, Pena MT, Choi SS, Zalzal GH. Retained ventilation tubes: should they be removed at 2 years? Arch Otolaryngol Head Neck Surg. 2002;128:1357–60.

80. Hekkenberg RJ, Smitheringale AJ. Gelfoam/Gelfilm patching following the removal of ventilation tubes. J Otolaryngology. 1995;24:362–3.

81. Syms CA, Gould AR, Zeiders JW, Faw KD. Automated tube deployment: success demonstrated in OR. Otolaryngol Head Neck Surg. 2011;145:P51.

82. Gan CW, Chooi Wh, Ng HC, Wong YS, Venkatraman SS, Lim LH. Development of a novel biodegradable drug-eluting ventilation tube for chronic otitis media with effusion. Laryngoscope. 2013;123(7):1770–7.

83. Poe DS, Silvola J, Pyykko I. Balloon dilation of the cartilaginous Eustachian tube. Otolaryngol Head Neck Surg. 2011;144(4):563–9.

Management of Chronic Suppurative Otitis Media

Sarah Prunty, Jennifer Ha and Shyan Vijayasekaran

Definition of CSOM

Chronic suppurative otitis media (CSOM) is one of the most common preventable causes of acquired hearing loss in children and is more prevalent in developing nations, where suppurative complications have a significant impact on childhood mortality. As such CSOM contributes to a significant global health burden. The definition of CSOM is chronic inflammation of the middle ear cleft (MEC), in the presence of a non-intact tympanic membrane that leads to frequent and recurrent otorrhea from the ear [1]. There has been a lack of consensus regarding the duration of symptoms. The World Health Organization (WHO) definition is a discharging ear that persists beyond 2 weeks but many otolaryngologists would say that acute otitis media (AOM) transitions to CSOM after at least 6 weeks of otorrhea and despite medical treatment [2–4]. In addition, certain specialists will refer to active and inactive disease. The term active CSOM is used to refer to perforation associated with infection whereas a chronic perforation in the absence of infection is termed inactive disease [5]. The ear can subsequently become reinfected by reflux of bacteria from the nasopharynx or from the introduction of pathogens from the external ear canal.

S. Vijayasekaran (✉) · S. Prunty · J. Ha
Department of Otolaryngology Head and Neck Surgery, Perth Children's Hospital, 6/1 Salvado Road, E6008 Subiaco, WA, Australia

Epidemiology of CSOM

True prevalence and incidence of CSOM is difficult to establish given the wide range of definitions for the condition. The WHO estimates the global burden of illness as a result of CSOM to include 65–330 million people worldwide. Approximately 60% of these individuals suffer significant hearing impairment and 28,000 die, usually as a complication of the disease. Ninety percent of CSOM occurs in South East Asia and the Western Pacific as well as certain parts of Africa [1]. A 4% prevalence rate of CSOM is considered to be indicative of a major public health issue [6]. Indigenous populations such as Inuit from Alaska, Canada and Greenland, American Indians and Australian Aboriginals are considered especially high risk. Among Australian Aboriginals, as many as 50% of the children suffer from CSOM [7]. These startlingly high prevalence rates are thought to be multifactorial in etiology but environmental factors are likely to be most strongly implicated. Young Aboriginal children have been shown to suffer early exposure to OM pathogens, persistent bacterial colonization, and chronic mucosal disease [8]. CSOM is generally thought to occur secondary to an episode of AOM in childhood but may also occur as a sequel of otitis media with effusion (OME) [5]. Risk factors for AOM are most likely implicated in the prognosis and development of CSOM: age, race, frequent upper respiratory tract infection, poor access to health care, crowded living conditions, poor hygiene and nutrition, attendance

D. Preciado (ed.), *Otitis Media: State of the art concepts and treatment*, DOI 10.1007/978-3-319-17888-2_12

at day care centers, bottle-feeding [9], exposure to passive smoking [10], and family history of OM. CSOM is least prevalent in developed nations such as the USA and European countries and when it occurs it is usually linked to tympanostomy tube (TT) insertion [11]. Placement of TTs can be associated with CSOM. One meta-analysis showed the rate of chronic otorrhea in intubated ears was 3.8%, recurrent otorrhea was 7.4%, and both of these sequelae were associated with longer-term TTs [12].

Genetics of CSOM

Even though the genetics of CSOM is poorly understood there are several studies looking at the genetics of AOM and COME. These include epidemiological studies of various methodologies as well as genetic studies [13–15]. Candidate gene studies have identified a handful of genes contributing to OM susceptibility, including several immune genes, such as *IL10* and *TNF*, as well as *FBXO11*, which have been significantly associated with OM in three independent cohorts [16–18]. The first genome-wide association study looking at the OM phenotype has identified *CAPN14* and *GALNT14* on chromosome 2p23.1 and the *BPIFA* gene cluster on chromosome 20q11.21 as novel candidate genes which warrant further analysis [19].

Microbiology of CSOM

OM occurs when viruses and bacteria evade the host mucociliary and immune responses establishing inflammation within the middle ear (ME) [20]. Chronic infection is often polymicrobial in nature with *Pseudomonas aeruginosa* and *Staphylococcus aureus* being the most common organisms isolated. Other isolates include *Staphylococcus epidermis*, *Proteus* species, beta-hemolytic *Streptococcus*, *Haemophilus influenza*, and enteric Gram-negative *bacilli* [21–23]. In recent years, the importance of the role of bacterial biofilm has come to light in the pathogenesis of CSOM, particularly in relation to the place-

ment of TTs. Van Leeuwenhoek first described bacterial biofilm in the seventeenth century when he examined the "animalcules" on the surface of his own teeth. Costerton and his colleagues put the modern theory of biofilm predominance forward in 1978 [24]. This theory has subsequently been refined to a community of bacteria irreversibly adherent to a surface, embedded in a self-produced matrix of extracellular polymeric substance, and exhibits altered phenotype with respect to the growth rate and gene transcription [25]. Biofilm and intracellular infection have been demonstrated on ME mucosa of children with CSOM, recurrent AOM, and chronic OME, and are mechanisms of bacterial persistence in the ME causing recalcitrance to treatment and disease recurrence [26–28]. Similarly, a number of studies have shown that TTs are highly subject to biofilm build up [29] which leads to refractory otorrhea and TT occlusion. Systemic antibiotics are known to have poor ME biofilm penetration. Krause et al. investigated the concentrations of a number of antimicrobial agents in ME fluid. For all agents it was shown that ME concentrations were significantly lower than serum concentrations [30]. A number of studies have been conducted looking at the use of TTs with resistance to biofilm formation with some promise. Phosphorylcholine-coated fluoroplastic TTs have been demonstrated to inhibit biofilm formation by both *P. aeruginosa* and *S. aureus* [31].

Management of CSOM

The management of CSOM has two principal aims: First, to eradicate infection and hence reduce morbidity and mortality, second, to close the tympanic membrane perforation to reduce hearing loss and risk of reinfection of the ME [1]. Recognition of those cases that are better managed surgically should be prompt to avoid delayed treatment and reduce morbidity. In some cases, this means instituting treatment to stop discharge from the ear before it can be established whether the patient has either active mucosal chronic otitis media (COM) or active squamous

COM (cholesteatoma) both of which require surgical intervention [32].

Nonsurgical

Medical management of CSOM is appropriate in the absence of cholesteatomatous disease, atticoantral disease, or suppurative complications of OM. There is a general lack of consensus among physicians regarding the optimal medical management of CSOM. A number of Cochrane review studies have examined the benefits of aural toilet, topical antiseptics, topical antimicrobials, systemic antimicrobials (oral and parenteral), and topical and systemic steroids. Presently, aural toilet combined with topical antibiotics is the mainstay therapy [1]. Quinolone antibiotics are the most commonly used topical agents but there are not many studies comparing agents. One randomized controlled trial (RCT) compared topical ciprofloxacin (CIP) with topical framycetin-gramicidin-dexamethasone (FGD) for the treatment of CSOM in Australian Aboriginal children. The study showed similar rates of improvement for both treatment arms (70 % CIP vs. 72 % FGD; CI-20–16) [33]. Topical quinolones are generally favored over nonquinolones because of the lack of safety data for the latter. The above trial did not show any significant difference in conductive hearing loss for CIP versus FGD, nor did it show the development of sensorineural loss, but ototoxicity was not an outcome that was directly measured in the study. Topical quinolones have been shown to be more effective than systemic quinolones in treating ear discharge at 1–2 weeks [34]. A Cochrane review has shown that topical antibiotics alone are better than systemic antibiotics in terms of resolution of otorrhea and eradication of ME bacteria [1]. A similar review in 2009 looked at whether combined topical and systemic antibiotics are better than topical antibiotics alone [34]. It found no trials showing statistically significant benefit from the addition of systemic antibiotics to topical treatment despite an increase in the cost of treatment and adverse effects of oral therapy. Leach et al. investigated the benefit of prophylactic antibiotics in relation to AOM and CSOM. They concluded that there is still uncertainty about the impact of prophylactic antibiotics on episodic AOM with perforation and CSOM [35].

For some patients otorrhea will persist despite aggressive aural toilet and prolonged courses of topical antibiotics. For these patients a long-term course (6–8 weeks) of parenteral antimicrobial therapy should be considered. Appropriate agents depend on culture results but generally include penicillin with anti-Pseudomonal cover such as piperacillin or a third-generation cephalosporin such as ceftazidime. Many of these patients will require tympanomastoid surgery.

Surgical

Surgery is indicated in cases of CSOM that are refractory to maximal medical therapy. There are several aims of surgery but the most important by far is to achieve a safe and dry ear [36]. Secondary considerations include stopping the discharge, healing the tympanic membrane, and restoring function to the ear [32]. Tympanoplasty, with or without mastoidectomy, is the primary procedure performed. Tympanoplasty is an operation to eradicate disease in the ME and reconstruct the hearing mechanism with or without using a graft to recreate the tympanic membrane [37]. Many materials have been used as graft material, the most popular of which is temporalis fascia, first described in the 1960s, [38] because it is easily harvested at the time of surgery and closely resembles the innate structure. Other grafts used include perichondrium, cartilage (tragus or conchal bowl), fat, vein, periosteum, and even Alloderm [39]. Three approaches are used in tympanoplasty: transcanal, endaural, or postauricular. The decision to use a particular approach is based on the size and location of the perforation, individual patient anatomy, and surgeon preference. Grafts may be placed medial or lateral to the tympanic membrane remnant depending on the location of the perforation and also the technical skills of the surgeon.

Mastoidectomy involves the removal of mastoid air cells, granulation tissue, and debris to eradicate infection and improved aeration of the ME. Mastoidectomy may be performed in conjunction with tympanoplasty either as a staged procedure or as a single surgery. The main relative indications for mastoidectomy in chronic ear disease include intractable otorrhea with chronic infection of the mastoid air cells, acquired cholesteatoma, previous failed tympanoplasty, and severe tympanic membrane retraction [36]. Mastoidectomy nomenclature can be confusing. An intact canal wall mastoidectomy or a canal-wall-up procedure preserves the bony superior and posterior canal walls while allowing removal of the mastoid cortex and air cells lateral to the facial nerve and optic capsule. A canal-wall-down or open cavity procedure, which includes both modified radical and radical mastoidectomy, involves the removal of the superior and posterior external auditory ear canal walls in association with meatoplasty to create an open cavity. In a modified radical mastoidectomy, the ME is grafted whereas in a radical mastoidectomy, there is no attempt at reconstruction and a mastoid cavity is formed [40]. This allows maximal aeration of the mastoid and long-term monitoring for disease recurrence. The latter procedure is usually indicated in cases of recurrent cholesteatoma, only hearing ear, sclerotic mastoid, involvement of the posterior canal wall, the presence of fistula, in noncompliant patients or patients that are unfit for a second look procedure. Open cavity techniques are associated with reduced hearing [41].

There is controversy over the optimal time to perform tympanoplasty in children. Koch and colleagues advocate a higher success rate when surgery is performed after 8 years of age. While successful results are not impossible in children prior to this age, eustachian tube dysfunction and frequent upper respiratory tract infections cause many tympanoplasties to fail [42]. Mishiro retrospectively looked at whether mastoidectomy at the time of tympanoplasty influenced graft success rates. They found that success rates were similar in both groups (90.5 % in tympanoplasty with mastoidectomy vs. 93.3 % in tympanoplasty alone). Effectiveness of surgery seems more dependent on patient selection and timing of surgery [43]. One study showed that tympano-

mastoidectomy for CSOM without cholesteatoma eradicated infection in 92 % of the cases. Poorer outcomes were associated with resistant strains of *P. aeruginosa*. Postoperative air-bone gap of 20 dB was achieved in only 62 % of the patients [44]. A meta-analysis done by Vrabec showed that surgical technique, prior adenoidectomy, presence of active infection, size of perforation, status of the contralateral ear, and eustachian tube function may not predict better healing [45].

Future Directions

The future directions of research are mainly aimed at prevention of CSOM in high-risk populations. Many studies are targeting biofilm as a means of an attempt to reduce the burden of disease caused by CSOM. One study in Western Australia is looking at using dornase alfa, a drug used in cystic fibrosis to reduce viscosity of secretions and shown to improve lung function, at the time of TT insertion to breakdown neutrophil extracellular traps (NETS), which harbor live bacteria and biofilm [46]. Dornase alfa may be a useful adjunct treatment in recurrent or chronic OM. Directly degrading the DNA may improve bacterial clearance from the ME by reducing biofilm stability and causing bacteria to return to their planktonic form which are more susceptible to locally (or systemically) administered antimicrobials and host immune mechanisms. Other targets include looking at vaccination against the primary pathogens of OM. The heptavalent PCV vaccine against *Streptococcus pneumoniae* has been shown to provide some protection against OM while significantly reducing frequency of medical presentations and need for TT placement in affluent populations [47]. However there is little evidence to suggest a reduction in CSOM and this is especially the case in high-risk groups such as the North American and Australian indigenous populations. This may be partially due to replacement of OM disease by non-vaccine serotypes and *H. influenzae*. The outcomes use of a 10-valent pneumococcal Haemophilus protein D conjugate vaccine and a 13-valent PCV that target these two groups of pathogens is much anticipated [48].

New surgical techniques, such as the use of b-FGF (fibroblast growth factor) on gelatin sponge held in position by fibrin glue, which can be highly successful at treating even large perforations, are also currently being investigated [49].

References

1. Acuin J. Chronic suppurative otitis media—burden of illness and management options. Geneva: WHO; 2004.
2. Roland PS. Chronic suppurative otitis media: a clinical overview. Ear Nose Throat J. 2002;81(8):8–10.
3. Verhoeff M, van der Veen EL, Rovers MM, Sanders EA, Schilder AG. Chronic suppurative otitis media: a review. Int J Paediatr Otorhinolaryngol. 2005;70:1–12.
4. Leiberman A, Fliss DM, Dagan R. Medical treatment of chronic suppurative otitis media without cholesteatoma in children—a two-year follow-up. Int J Paediatr Otorhinolaryngol. 1992;24:25–33.
5. Bluestone CD. Epidemiology and pathogenesis of CSOM: implications for prevention and treatment. Int J Paediatr Otorhinolaryngol. 1998;42(3):207–23.
6. 1996 W. Prevention of hearing impairment from chronic Otitis media. 1996.
7. Harvey J, Coates PSM, Leach AJ, Couzos S. Otitis media in Aboriginal children: tackling a major health problem. Med J Aust. 2002;177(4):177–8.
8. Coates HJ. Chronic suppurative otitis media in indigenous populations: the Australian Aborigine. Ear Nose Throat J. 2002;81(8):11–2.
9. Wintermeyer SM, Nahata M. Chronic suppurative otitis media. Ann Pharmacother. 1994;28(111):2–9.
10. Adair-Bischoff CE, Sauve R. Environmental tobacco smoke in middle ear disease in pre-school age children. Arch Pediatr Adolesc Med. 1998;152(2):127–33.
11. van der Veen EL, Schilder AG, van Heerbeek N, Verhoeff M, Zielhuis GA, Rovers MM. Predictors of chronic suppurative otitis media in children. Arch Otolaryngol Head Neck Surg. 2006;132:1115–8.
12. Kay DJ, Nelson M, Rosenfeld RM. Meta-analysis of tympanostomy tube sequelae. Otolaryngol Head Neck Surg. 2001;124(4):374–80. (Brooklyn, New York)
13. Kvaerner KJ, Tambs K, Harris JR, Magnus P. Distribution and heritability of recurrent ear infections. Annals Otol Rhinol Laryngol. 1997;106(8):624–32.
14. Rye MS, Blackwell JM, Jamieson SE. Genetic susceptibility to otitis media in childhood. Laryngoscope. 2012;122(3):665–75.
15. Casselbrant ML, Mandel EM, Fall PA, Rockette HE, Kurs-Lasky M, Bluestone CD, Ferrell RE. The heritability of otitis media: a twin and triplet study. JAMA. 1999;282(22):2125–30.
16. Segade F, Daly KA, Allred D, Hicks PJ, Cox M, Brown M, Hardisty-Hughes RE, Brown SD, Rich SS, Bowden DW. Association of the FBXO11 gene with COME/ROM in the Minnesota COME/ROM family study. Arch Otolaryngol Head Neck Surg. 2006;132(7):729–33.
17. Rye MS, Wiertsema SP, Scaman ES, Oommen J, Sun W, Francis RW, Ang W, Pennell CE, Burgner D, Richmond P, Vijayasekaran S, Coates HL, Brown SD, Blackwell JM, Jamieson SE. FBXO11, a regulator of the TGFb pathway, is associated with severe otitis media in Western Australian children. Genes Immun. 2011;12:352–9.
18. Rye MS, Blackwell JM, Jamieson SE. Genetic susceptibility to otitis media in childhood. Laryngoscope. 2012;122(3):665–75.
19. Rye MS, Warrington NM, Scaman ES, Vijayasekaran S, Coates HL, Anderson D, Pennell CE, Blackwell JM, Jamieson SE. Genome-wide association study to identify the genetic determinants of otitis media susceptibility in childhood. PLoS ONE. 2012;7(10):e48215.
20. Massa HM CA, Lehmann D. Otitis media: viruses, bacteria, biofilms and vaccines. Med J Aust. 2009;191 (9 Suppl):S44–9.
21. Induharan R. Antibiotics in chronic suppurative otitis media: a bacteriologic study. Ann Otol Rhinol Laryngol. 1999;108(5):440–5.
22. Fliss DM. Aerobic bacteriology of chronic suppurative otitis media without cholesteatoma in children. Ann Otol Rhinol Laryngol. 1992;101:866–9.
23. Margaret A. Kenna CB. Microbiology of chronic suppurative otitis media in children. Pediatr Infect Dis. 1986;86:223–5.
24. Costerton JW, Geesey G, Cheng KJ. How bacteria stick. Sci Am. 1978;238(1):86–95.
25. Donlan RM, Costerton JW. Biofilms: survival mechanisms of clinically relevant microorganisms. Clin Microbiol Rev. 2002;15(2):167–93.
26. Coates H, Langlands J, Filion P, Keil AD, et al. The role of chronic infection in children with otitis media with effusion: evidence for intracellular persistence of bacteria. Otolaryngol Head Neck Surg. 2008;138:778–81.
27. Ruth BT, Rigby PJ, Selma PW, Filion P, Langlands J, Harvey LC, Vijayasekaran S, Keil AD, Richmond PC. Multi-species bacterial biofilm and intracellular infection in otitis media. BMC Pediatr. 2011;11:94. (1996, WHO)
28. Hall-Stoodley L, Hu FZ, Gieseke A, Nistico L, Nguyen D, Hayes J, Forbes M, Greenberg DP, Dice B, Burrows A, Wackym PA, Stoodley P, Post JC, Ehrlich GD, Kerschner JE. Direct detection of bacterial biofilms on the middle-ear mucosa of children with chronic otitis media. JAMA. 2006;296(2):202–11.
29. Barakate M, Becknham E, Curotta J, Da Cruz M. Bacterial biofilm adherence to middle-ear ventilation

tubes: scanning electron micrograph images and literature review. J Laryngol Otol. 2007;121:993–7.

30. Krause PJ, Owens NJ, Nightingale CH, Kilmek JJ, Lehmann WB, Quintillani R. Penetration of amoxicillin, cefaclor, erythromycin-sulfisoxazole, and trimethoprim-sulfamethoxazole into the middle ear fluid of patients with chronic serous otitis media. J Infect Dis. 1982;145(6):815–21.

31. Berry JA, Biedlingmaier JF, Whelan PJ. In vitro resistance to bacterial biofilm formation on coated fluoroplastic tympanostomy tubes. Otolaryngol Head Neck Surg. 2000;123:246–51.

32. Acuin JM, Chiong C, Yang N. Surgery for chronically discharging ears with underlying eardrum perforations. Cochrane Database. 2009.

33. Leach A, Wood Y, Gadil E, Stubbs E, Morris P. Topical ciprofloxin versus topical framycetin-gramicidin-dexamethasone in Australian Aboriginal children with recently treated chronic suppurative otitis media a randomized controlled trial. Pediatr Infect Dis J. 2008;27(8):692–8.

34. Macfadyen CA, Acuin JM, Gamble CL. Systemic antibiotics versus topical treatments for chronically discharging ears with underlying eardrum perforations (Review). Cochrane Database. 2009.

35. Leach AJ, Morris PS. Antibiotics for the prevention of acute and chronic suppurative otitis media in children (Review). Cochrane Database. 2006.

36. Haynes DS. Surgery for chronic ear disease. Ear Nose Throat J. 2001;80(6):S8–11.

37. Otolaryngology. The committee on conservation of hearing of the American academy of opthalmology and otolaryngology. Standard classification for surgery of chronic ear infection. Arch Otolaryngol Head Neck Surg. 1965;81:204–205.

38. Storrs LA. Myringoplasty with the use of fascia grafts. Arch Otolaryngol Head Neck Surg. 1961;71:45–9.

39. Haynes DS, Vos JD, Labadie RF. Acellular allograft dermal matrix for tympanoplasty. Curr Opin Otolaryngol Head Neck Surg. 2006;13(5):283–6.

40. Bennett M, Warren F, Haynes D. Indications and technique in mastoidectomy. Otolaryngol Clin North Am. 2006;39:1095–113.

41. Stankovic MD. Audiologic results of surgery for cholesteatoma: short- and long-term follow up of influential factors. Otolo Neurotol. 2008;29:933.

42. Koch WM. Tympanoplasty in children. The Boston Children's Hospital experience. Arch Otolaryngol Head Neck Surg. 1990;116:35–40.

43. Mishiro Y, Sakagami M, Takahashi Y, Kitahara T, Kajikawa H, Kubo T. Tympanoplasty with and without mastoidectomy for non-cholesteatomatous chronic otitis media. Eur Arch Otorhinolaryngol. 2001;258(1):13–5.

44. Vartiainen E. Tympanomastoidectomy for chronic otitis media without cholesteatoma. Otolaryngol Head Neck Surg. 1992;106(3):230–4.

45. Vrabec JT, Deskin RW, Grady JJ. Meta-analysis of pediatric tympanoplasty. Arch Otolaryngol Head Neck Surg. 1999;125(5):530–4.

46. Thornton RB, Wiertsema SP, Kirkham LA, Rigby PJ, Vijayasekaran S, Coates HL, Richmond PC. Neutrophil extracellular traps and bacterial biofilms in middle ear effusion of children with recurrent acute Otitis media—a potential treatment target. PLOS ONE. 2013;8(2):e53837.

47. Fireman F, Black SB, Shinefield HR, Lee J, Lewis E, Ray P. Impact of the pneumococcal conjugate vaccine on otitis media. Pediatr Infect Dis. 2003;22(1):10–7.

48. Mackenzie GA, Carapetis JR, Leach AJ, Morris PS. Pneumococcal vaccination and otitis media in Australian Aboriginal infants: comparison of two birth cohorts before and after introduction of vaccination. BioMed Central. 2009;19:14.

49. Kanemaru S, Umeda H, Kitani Y, Nakamura T, Hirano S, Ito J. Regenerative treatment for tympanic membrane perforation. J Otol Neurotol. 2011;32(8):1218–23.

Otitis Media Complications

13

José San Martín and Ximena Fonseca

List of Abbreviations

AM	Acute mastoiditis
AOM	Acute otitis media
COM	Chronic otitis media
CT	Computed tomography
EOMC	Extracranial otitis media complications
FP	Facial palsy
IOMC	Intracranial otitis media complications
IV	Intravenous
LST	Lateral sinus thrombosis
MR	Magnetic resonance
OM	Otitis media
OMC	Otitis media complications
OME	Otitis media with effusion
PCV7	Heptavalent pneumococcal conjugate vaccine
SA	Subperiosteal abscess

Incidence and Classification

Acute otitis media (AOM) is a very frequent condition in children, especially in males under 3 years of age. Currently, in the post-antibiotic era, complications from AOM are very unusual.

Regarding the incidence of complications of otitis media (OMC), some literature has reported an increasing incidence [1, 2], but most of the recent papers report that the incidence has not increased [3–5]. It would be interesting to analyze if the modifications of the treatments suggested by the different guidelines for AOM used in America and European countries (among others), the use of vaccines, and the changes in susceptibility of the involved bacteria are impacting the incidence of complications. Paradoxically, it seems that reduction of antibiotic use in AOM could have a beneficial role in children with complications, as shown by a recent publication [6] that reported that 94 % of the bacteria found in AOM complications are susceptible to penicillin.

Otitis media complications can result from AOM or chronic otitis media (COM) with or without cholesteatoma. Yet, most of the cases are secondary to AOM. A meta-analysis published by Rosenfeld estimated an OM complication incidence of 0.12–0.24 % of AOM cases [7].

Otitis media complications can be classified as extracranial (EOMC), intracranial (IOMC), or both.

Factors involved in the development of these complications can be related to the pathogen, for example, bacterial virulence or the presence of resistant pneumococcus and others related to the patient as systemic or local immune deficiencies, allowing dissemination through areas of less resistance or from sequestered infections.

J. San Martín (✉) · X. Fonseca
Department of Otolaryngology, Head and Neck Surgery, Hospital Clinico Pontificia Universidad Catolica De Chile, Marcoleta 350, Piso 2, Santiago 8330033, Chile
e-mail: jsanmart@uc.cl

X. Fonseca
e-mail: mxfonsecaa@gmail.com

© Springer International Publishing Switzerland 2015
D. Preciado (ed.), *Otitis Media: State of the art concepts and treatment*, DOI 10.1007/978-3-319-17888-2_13

123

Extracranial Complications

Acute Mastoiditis

Acute mastoiditis (AM) is inflammation of the air cells of the mastoid due to the extension of the infection from the middle ear. It is the most frequent complication of AOM. The incidence of AM in children with AOM is 0.24–0.74% [8] and is more frequent among children 2 years of age or younger. Anthonsen [6] found that 72% of children with AM were 2 years or less and the incidence of AM in children was 4.8/100,000 children. Other authors report an incidence of 11–16.8/100,000 in children less than 2 years and 4.3–7.1/100,000 in older than 2 years [3]. The general incidence reported in the group between 0 and 14 years is 1.2–6.1/100,000 children [5].

Concerns regarding an increase in AM due to the restriction in the use of antibiotics suggested by guidelines have been ruled out by several authors that have compared the incidence of complications along the years [3, 6, 9].

When the extension of the infection from the middle ear gets to the mastoid, it produces a periostitis that can lead to the destruction or lysis of the bony trabeculae of the mastoid, in turn leading to coalescence of the air cells, and resulting in AM.

It is important to mention that during an inflammatory process such as noncomplicated AOM or otitis media with effusion (OME), opacification of the mastoid cells can be seen in radiologic exams, but if there is no lysis of the opacified air cells and coalescence of them, the diagnosis of AM is not correct [10]. When the infection in the mastoid compromises the integrity of the cortical layer of the mastoid, a subperiosteal abscess (SA) results. The most frequent location is retroauricular, less frequent is a Bezold's abscess where the infection propagates to the tip of the mastoid and Citelli's abscess where the extension is towards the occipital region [11].

In terms of the clinical presentation, in around half of the cases AM is the first manifestation of the middle-ear infection, with no clinical history of actual or recent AOM [1, 3, 12].

A retrospective study in Denmark found that 100% of children with AM had ear protrusion, whereas retroauricular edema and redness were present in around 95% of cases (Fig. 13.1). Other symptoms included retroauricular tenderness in 85%, external auditory canal edema in 43%, retroauricular abscess in 32%, and facial paralysis in 6% of cases [6].

As mentioned, the use of antibiotics in AOM does not appear to prevent complications. Anthonsen [6] reports that 35% of children with AM were under antibiotics at the moment of the complication and there was no difference in the development of an abscess among children receiving or not the antibiotic (odds ratio 0.97). Similarly, Leskinen in Finland [13] reported that 55% of children with AM were receiving antibiotics when admitted to hospital. They found no correlation between the prior intake of antibiotics and the percentage of mastoidectomies that had to be performed for AM. Other authors record that 85% of patients were under antibiotic coverage [14].

The clinical evaluation of a child with an OMC should include an assessment of the general and neurological condition of the child, the presence of fever and lethargy, search for facial palsy, and signs suggesting an elevation of intracranial pressure. A thorough otomicroscopic exam should be done and, if possible, audiometry and tympanometry.

The bacteriology of AM is variable with the most frequent bacteria recovered being *Strep-*

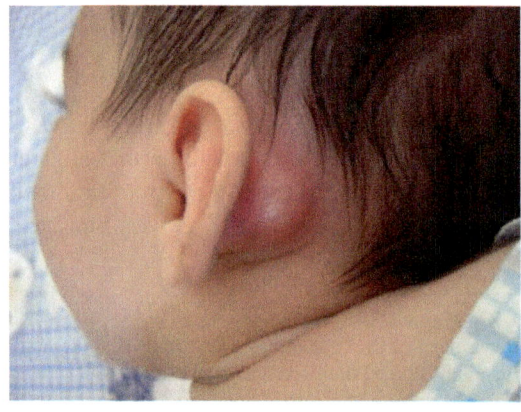

Fig. 13.1 Note the ear protrusion, retroauricular edema, and redness in this patient with acute mastoiditis and subperiosteal abscess

tococcus pneumoniae (25–51%), *S. pyogenes* (2–26%), *Pseudomonas aeruginosa* (4.5–29%), *Haemophilus influenzae* (4.5–16%), *Staphylococcus aureus* (3.5–8%) and *Fusobacterium necrophorum* (5.8%) [1, 8, 11, 15].

Radiological imaging in AM shows an occupation by secretions of the middle ear and mastoid cells associated with coalescence (Fig. 13.2). Some papers mention that routine computed tomography (CT) is not justified for AM [16], and that CT should only be done on the basis of the clinical presentation of each patient. Others do not agree [17], arguing that patients with AM and concomitant intracranial complications are often indistinguishable from noncomplicated AM patients. This makes CT a helpful tool in diagnosis, although there is no consensus in terms of whether it is mandatory in all cases of AM. Regardless, high-resolution temporal bone and brain CT carry a sensibility of 97% and a positive predictive value of 94% in the diagnosis of an intracranial complication of AM [18].

The prognosis of AM is closely linked to the presence of intracranial complications; hence, high clinical suspicion, early diagnosis, and appropriate treatment are necessary.

There are some controversies regarding the treatment of AM. For some groups, surgical treatment should be done upon AM diagnosis, with a simple mastoidectomy, for others management can be more conservative consisting of intravenous (IV) antibiotics or IV antibiotics and myringotomy with or without tube placement. Psarommatis [19] in a retrospective study of 155 patients with AM proposes an algorithm for its management. According to him, patients should be divided into three groups, one of patients with AM and suspicion of intracranial complication, another with isolated AM, and the third with AM and SA. According to his algorithm all the groups should be managed with myringotomy and IV antibiotics in the form of a third-generation cephalosporin (cefotaxime or ceftriaxone) and clindamycin. In patients with SA, a percutaneous drainage of it is done by aspiration or incision. If an intracranial complication is suspected, the radiologic evaluation is mandatory and if it is positive, a simple mastoidectomy should be done immediately. After initial management, all patients without a favorable response after 3–5 days should receive a simple mastoidectomy. Upon discharge, oral antibiotics should be prescribed for 7–10 days, with the exception of patients with intracranial complications that should receive oral antibiotics for at least 15 days.

Other authors recommend a similar management, proposing a more conservative treatment of noncomplicated AM following AOM, including IV antibiotics, myringotomy (with or without tympanosotomy tubes), and percutaneous drainage of possible SA [16, 20, 21] Groth reports that previous mastoidectomy seems to predispose the patient to recurrent AM. This could suggest a more conservative therapy [22].

In cases of AM in patients with COM with or without cholesteatoma, there is consensus that a mastoidectomy with removal of granulations and cholesteatoma should be done as soon as possible and antibiotics must include coverage for *S. aureus and P. aeruginosa*.

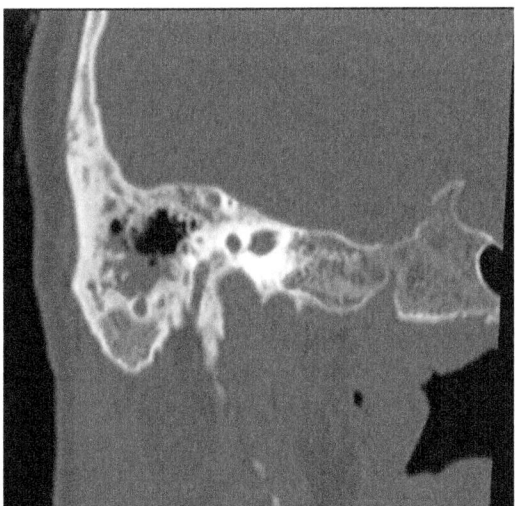

Fig. 13.2 Computed tomography showing occupation by secretions of the mastoid cells, associated to coalescent erosion of them

Facial Palsy

Facial palsy (FP) due to otitis remains infrequent, with a reported incidence of 0.005% in AOM [23]

and from 0.16 to 5.1 % in COM [24]. FP in AOM occurs usually after inflammation of the horizontal segment (tympanic) of the nerve, where it crosses the middle ear. In patients without chronic middle-ear disease, FP is usually secondary to neuropraxis from edema and nerve compression and/or bacterial toxic metabolites [25].

The House-Brackmann classification describes the degree of FP in each patient. There are six categories, I (normal function), II (mild paresis), III (moderate paresis), IV (moderate to severe paresis), V (severe paresis) and VI (complete palsy) [26].

CT scanning is indicated in patients that do not have a favorable evolution of FP or in cases in which there is a suspicion of a coexistent complication or in cases with a precedent of COM [24].

The use of magnetic resonance (MR) with gadolinium excludes other causes of FP. MR can show the inflammation of the nerve but does not determine the severity of the lesion [25].

Treatment includes wide-spectrum antibiotics with coverage for *Streptococci, H. influenzae,* and *Staphylococci* and tympanocentesis (for gram and culture) and myringotomy with tubes [27], although some authors recommend tubes only in cases with recurrent AOM or OME [25]. This conservative management in patients with less severe palsy (House–Brackmann II–III) is supported by the remission of symptoms in almost all the patients treated [23, 28]. Given the high rate of spontaneous recovery of FP, electrophysiological studies are not indicated for mild cases. In case of more severe FP (House–Brackmann IV–VI), electrophysiological tests, such as nervous excitability, maximal excitability electromyography, and electroneurography, can be helpful. The more severe degeneration of the nerve correlates with a bad recovery prognosis and may indicate surgical mastoidectomy with facial nerve decompression [25]. There is no consensus about the moment to perform surgery. Although some authors suggest it should be done during the acute phase, others suggest medical treatment and mastoidectomy should be performed and decompression should be postponed [29–31].

Complete facial palsy as a complication from AM or COM must be treated surgically. If it is due to an AM, mastoidectomy and myringotomy with a tube is suggested, if it is due to a COM, surgery must be done immediately, removing the cholesteatoma and granulation tissue [32, 33], as this situation may be associated to a poor prognosis [34].

Labyrinthitis

Labyrinthine infection results from extension of the infection from the middle-ear space to the cochlea and/or the vestibular system. Generally, the dissemination is via the round window, although it can also occur through the oval window, a perilymphatic fistula, or defects secondary to chronic infection with or without cholesteatoma, trauma, or postsurgical defects [25]. Labyrinthitis can be classified as serous and suppurative, with serous being far more frequent. It is produced by the action of toxins and inflammatory mediators without frank bacterial invasion into the inner ear. Cochlear involvement is more frequent than vestibular involvement. Labyrinthitis should be suspected in cases of AOM with sudden SNHL and/or vertigo [25]. If labyrinthitis occurs chronically in patients with COM, high-frequency SNHL is more likely, given usual greater damage of the basal turn of the cochlea [25].

Suppurative labyrinthitis is very infrequent, comprising approximately 2 % of the intratemporal complications of AOM [35]. It results from frank bacterial invasion into the inner ear and is highly suggestive of anatomical defects or immune deficiencies [25]. Clinical presentation is more severe, with high fever, vertigo, ear pain, nausea, vomiting, sweating, severe SNHL, and spontaneous nystagmus towards the unaffected ear. Any child with AOM and with nystagmus and vertigo should be treated aggressively because this suppurative labyrinthitis can progress to meningitis [25]. Although not mandatory for diagnosis, MR is the most sensitive imaging modality in the workup of labyrinthitis, showing an enhancement of the fluid in the labyrinth when gadolinium contrast is used. CT is only used as a presurgical study, looking for congenital anatomical anomalies, erosions, or cholesteatoma.

Treatment includes IV antibiotics with presumptive coverage for the most frequent pathogens in AOM *(S. pneumoniae, H. influenzae,* and *M. catarrhalis)*, along with early myringotomy with or without tympanostomy tube placement. In cases of precedent COM, the antibiotic coverage should include *S. aureus* and *P. aeruginosa* coverage. In cases of coalescent mastoiditis, suppurative COM or cholesteatoma, a mastoidectomy with removal of the tissue is involved, and repair of an eventual perilymphatic fistula must be done [25]. Patients with serous labyrinthitis generally present a rapid resolution of vertigo and hearing loss although some deficit can persist. In case of patients with suppurative labyrinthitis and severe SNHL, recovery is very infrequent. Vertigo can last for weeks or months, until it is successfully compensated by contralateral ear and central mechanisms [25]. Ossificant labyrinthitis is a complication that can occur after acute labyrinthitis, where the labyrinth is replaced by fibrous and/or bony tissue, with a loss of its function. This is more frequent after meningitis and suppurative meningococcal labyrinthitis, but can also occur in cases of suppurative labyrinthitis without associated meningitis.

Petrositis

Petrositis results from the extension of the infection from the tympanic cavity towards the petrous apex air cells. It is very infrequent, and generally occurs along with intracranial complications of OM [35]. The classic clinical presentation of petrositis is called the Gradenigo's triad: pain in trigeminal distribution, otorrhea, and VI nerve palsy. However, its presentation can be variable, the triad being present in only up to 40 % of patients [36]. An ear CT should be done if a destructive lesion of the petrous apex is suspected. If the lesion is confirmed, MR can give more information as well as show possible adjacent meningeal involvement. MR allows to differentiate among petrositis, cholesterol granuloma, cholesteatoma,

and neoplasms (schwannoma, meningioma, condroma, or chordoma) [36].

Bacteria usually recovered are *S. pneumoniae, H. influenzae* y *P. aeruginosa* [11]. Reports consisting of small-patient series recommend early wide-spectrum IVs antibiotic treatment along with myringotomy with tympanostomy tube insertion and mastoidectomy in refractory cases or those secondary to COM [37–39].

Intracranial Complications

Since the introduction of antibiotics in the twentieth century, the incidence of intracranial complications due to OM significantly decreased from 2.3 % to 0.24–0.04 % [40]. Although IOMC are far less frequent than EOMC, they are much more dangerous, with a reported mortality of 16–18 % [40, 41]. Around half of the patients have more than one complication simultaneously [40]. Acute meningitis and cerebral abscess are the most frequent IOMC [40, 42, 43]. Microbiology of the abscess is variable and is related to the underlying etiology of the complication (AOM vs. COM). In abscess secondary to AOM, *S. pneumoniae, S. pyogenes, S. aureus* y *H. influenzae* are cultured, in patients due to COM, *S. aureus, Proteus mirabilis, P. aeruginosa, Klebsiella* spp., *Enterococcus* and anaerobes are found [43–45].

When an IOMC is suspected, imaging a study is mandatory. High-resolution brain CT with contrast along with temporal CT is excellent for the diagnosis of OMC [18]. However, there is consensus that in these patients a brain MR with venography should also be done in order to evaluate the possibility of sigmoid sinus thrombosis or petrositis [45–47].

Acute Meningitis

As mentioned before, acute otogenic meningitis and cerebral abscess are the most frequent IOMC. Kangsanarak reported 51 % of meningitis and 42 % of cerebral abscess in a group of 43 patients with IOMC [40], Penido in a group of 33 patients with IOMC reported 46% of them presenting with cerebral abscess and 37% presenting with meningitis [43]. Lumbar puncture is usually performed if an acute meningitis is suspected but it is important to remember that this has to be performed after scanning to rule out elevated intracranial pressure, which could result in cerebral herniation or coning along with mortality during lumbar puncture [43]. Broad-spectrum intravenous antibiotics must be administered promptly along with myringotomy and ventilation tubes to obtain cultures and drainage of the middle ear. Mastoidectomy should be reserved for patients who do not respond to treatment within 48 h [48].

Intracranial Abscess

Otogenic intracranial abscess can be extradural, subdural, or parenchymatous. The most frequent locations are the temporal and cerebellar lobes [40, 41], with extradural ones being most frequent [44]. Although in adults these abscesses present in cases of underlying CSOM [40, 41, 49], in children these abscesses are more often seen in patients with AOM [42, 44]. They portend a high mortality rate (20–36%), especially in developing countries [40]. However, more recent studies in developed countries report a low mortality [42, 44]. The most frequent symptoms are fever and ear pain followed by headache and otorrea [44]. Altered mental status is more frequent in patients with subdural and intraparenchymatous abscesses than in extradural ones. Nausea, vomiting, diplopia, seizures, limb paresis, and meningeal signs can be found [44].

Most of the authors agree that treatment should include long-term broad-spectrum intravenous antibiotics with blood–brain barrier penetrance and the initial treatment should be modified and based on cultures and sensitivity as soon as possible. Several antibiotic treatments have been proposed, including combinations of third-generation cephalosporins, amoxicillin/clavulanic acid, ciprofloxacin, aminoglycosides, penicillin, vancomycin, metronidazole, chloramphenicol [40, 41, 45, 50], covering Gram positives, Gram negatives, S. aureus, anaerobic bacteria, and P. ae-

ruginosa. Regarding the surgical treatment there are some controversies. The standard accepted treatment is abscess drainage through trephination or excision through craniotomy followed by a differed otologic surgery of mastoid drainage. However, some authors recommend other treatments, such as combined early neurosurgery and mastoidectomy, mastoidectomy with evacuation of the abscess through the mastoidectomy; some groups even perform only the mastoidectomy and reserve the neurosurgery only for selected cases. All of these treatments are supported by reports of low and comparable morbidities and mortalities that have decreased, towards 0% [41, 43–45, 51–53]. Subdural abscess or empyema is an exception to this rule because it requires immediate neurosurgical drainage [41, 44, 50]. If the origin of the abscess is COM, mastoidectomy should be performed during the same hospitalization, either at the time of the neurosurgical procedure or after it. Mastoidectomy could be avoided only if the origin of the complication is AOM and if the patient has an excellent resolution with the initial treatment [43].

Lateral Sinus Thrombosis

Two-thirds of LST in children occur secondary to AOM and one-third to COM. Generally, it results from the erosion of the mastoid cortical bone adjacent to the sinus with subsequent infection of the peri-sinusal space. LST may also occur due to thrombophlebitis of the mastoid emissary veins without erosion of the contiguous cortical bone. In the past, this condition was associated with high mortality. After contemporary surgical intervention techniques along with antibiotic treatment, mortality, however, has decreased dramatically to around 1%. The most frequent symptoms and signs of LST are fever, headache, ear pain, vomiting, otorrhea, and cervical rigidity [54]. "Picket-fence fever pattern" described in pre-antibiotic era is infrequent nowadays [55]. Imaging study is very important for diagnosing this complication. Sensitivity of the MR (100%) and superior to contrast enhanced CT (87%) [54]. The most prevalent pathogens are group A

Streptococcus, S. pneumoniae, S. aureus, P. aeruginosa, and anaerobes [54]. The management of LST includes broad-spectrum antibiotics (vancomycine + third-generation cephalosporines + metronidazole) and prompt mastoid surgery with or without myringotomy with or without ventilation tubes. A simple mastoidectomy is indicated in cases of LST without cholesteatoma and a modified radical surgery should be performed in cases with cholesteatoma. Treatment of LST patients without mastoidectomy is also possible and could be considered in patients without intracranial abscess that are responding to broad-spectrum intravenous antibiotics [54]. Regarding the management of the thrombotic sinus, there are three possibilities: observation, needle aspiration, or thrombectomy, with a clear trend towards not evacuating the abscess given the risk of bleeding. Anticoagulation is given in most cases [54]. Ligation of the internal jugular vein is rarely done, reserved only for refractory sepsis, or septic lung embolism [54].

Changes in Post-vaccination Era

An important reduction in the incidence of invasive pneumococcal infections has been reported since the introduction of the heptavalent pneumococcal conjugate vaccine (PCV7). However, for AM specifically, PCV7 has not shown the same effect, and the incidence has remained stable or has in fact increased [56–59]. Halgrimson studied the incidence of AM in children younger than 2 years of age between 1999 and 2008; in 2001, before the widespread use of PCV7, the incidence was 11/100,000, in 2003, it dropped down to 4.5/100,000, and then it returned to 12/100,000 in 2008 [57]. On the other hand, *P. pneumoniae* is still the most frequent pathogen in cases of AM secondary to AOM. Choi et al. in his series reported the presence of *P. pneumoniae* in 34% of the cases in periods pre- and post-vaccination with PCV7 [58]. Halgrimson reported that in his series *P. pneumoniae* was responsible for 30% of the pathogens found in the pre-PCV7 and 50% in the post-PCV7 era [57]. Navazo-Eguía et al. reported that *P. pneumoniae* was isolated in 30%

of the cases in the pre-PCV7 era and in 42.1% in the post-vaccination era [59]. An increase in bacterial resistance has been found in *P. pneumoniae* isolated in AM post-PCV7. Halgrimson reported an increase in penicillin resistance from 0 to 38% comparing the pre- and post-PCV7 vaccination era [57]. Leibovitz in a revision in AM cases found an increase in the resistance to ceftriaxone from 7 to 30% [56]. Regarding the serotypes found in AM as well as in AOM, the serotypes included in the vaccine have been replaced by others not included in the vaccine, among which 19A is the most frequent. Ongkasuwan reports in his series that AM produced by 19A had an incidence of 0% in the pre-PCV7 era and 65.5% in the post-vaccine era [60]; these data are almost the same as the 65% reported by Giannakopoulos [14]. This serotype has been related to more severe cases of AM, with more sub-periostal abscess, as well as a greater antibiotic resistance [60]. Due to these findings and the introduction of the 13-valent pneumococcal conjugate vaccine, there must be a strict surveillance of the incidence of AM, the pathogens involved, and their resistance pattern.

References

1. Benito MB, Gorricho BP. Acute mastoiditis: increase in the incidence and complications. Int J Pediatr Otorhinolaryngol. 2007;71(7):1007–11.
2. Katz A, Leibovitz E, Greenberg D, Raiz S, Greenwald-Maimon M, Leiberman A, Dagan R. Acute mastoiditis in Southern Israel: a twelve year retrospective study (1990 through 2001). Pediatr Infect Dis J. 2003;22(10):878–82.
3. Kvaerner KJ, Bentdal Y, Karevold G. Acute mastoiditis in Norway: no evidence for an increase. Int J Pediatr Otorhinolaryngol. 2007;71(10):1579–83. Epub 2007 Aug 20.
4. Pritchett CV, Thorne MC. Incidence of pediatric acute mastoiditis: 1997–2006. Arch Otolaryngol Head Neck Surg. 2012;138(5):451–5.
5. Groth A, Enoksson F, Hermansson A, Hultcrantz M, Stalfors J, Stenfeldt K. Acute mastoiditis in children in Sweden 1993–2007—no increase after new guidelines. Int J Pediatr Otorhinolaryngol. 2011;75(12):1496–501.
6. Anthonsen K, Høstmark K, Hansen S, Andreasen K, Juhlin J, Homøe P, Caye-Thomasen P. Acute mastoiditis in children: a 10-year retrospective and validated multicenter study. Pediatr Infect Dis J. 2013;32(5):436–40.

7. Rosenfeld RM, Kay D. Natural history of untreated otitis media. In: Rosenfeld RM, Bluestone CD, editors. Evidence-based otitis media. Hamilton: BC Decker; 2003. p. 183–84.

8. Quesnel S, Nguyen M, Pierrot S, Contencin P, Manach Y, Couloigner V. Acute mastoiditis in children: a retrospective study of 188 patients. Int J Pediatr Otorhinolaryngol. 2010;74(12):1388–92.

9. Palma S, Fiumana E, Borgonzoni M, Bovo R, Rosignoli M, Martini A. Acute mastoiditis in children: the "Ferrara" experience. Int J Pediatr Otorhinolaryngol. 2007;71(11):1663–9.

10. Minks DP, Porte M, Jenkins N. Acute mastoiditis— he role of radiology. Clin Radiol. 2013;68(4):397–405. doi:10.1016/j.crad.2012.07.019. Epub 2012 Sep 11.

11. Leskinen K. Complications of acute otitis media in children. Curr Allergy Asthma Rep. 2005;5(4):308–12.

12. Groth A, Enoksson F, Hultcrantz M, Stalfors J, Stenfeldt K, Hermansson A. Acute mastoiditis in children aged 0–16 years—a national study of 678 cases in Sweden comparing different age groups. Int J Pediatr Otorhinolaryngol. 2012;76(10):1494–500.

13. Leskinen K, Jero J. Complications of acute otitis media in children in southern Finland. Int J Pediatr Otorhinolaryngol. 2004;68(3):317–24.

14. Giannakopoulos P, Chrysovergis A, Xirogianni A, Nikolopoulos TP, Radiotis A, Lebessi E, et al. Microbiology of acute mastoiditis and complicated or refractory acute otitis media among hospitalized children in the postvaccination era. Pediatr Infect Dis J. 2014;33(1):111–3.

15. Pang LH, Barakate MS, Havas TE. Mastoiditis in a paediatric population: a review of 11 years experience in management. Int J Pediatr Otorhinolaryngol. 2009;73(11):1520–4.

16. Tamir S, Schwartz Y, Peleg U, Perez R, Sichel JY. Acute mastoiditis in children: is computed tomography always necessary? Ann Otol Rhinol Laryngol. 2009;118:565–9.

17. Luntz M, Bartal K, Brodsky A, Shihada R. Acute mastoiditis: the role of imaging for identifying intracranial complications. Laryngoscope. 2012;122(12):2813–7.

18. Migirov L. Computed tomographic versus surgical findings in complicated acute otomastoiditis. Ann Otol Rhinol Laryngol. 2003;112(8):675–7.

19. Psarommatis IM, Voudouris C, Douros K, Giannakopoulos P, Bairamis T, Carabinos C. Algorithmic management of pediatric acute mastoiditis. Int J Pediatr Otorhinolaryngol. 2012;76(6):791–6.

20. Zanetti D, Nassif N. Indications for surgery in acute mastoiditis and their complications in children. Int J Pediatr Otorhinolaryngol. 2006;70(7):1175–82.

21. Bakhos D, Trijolet JP, Morinière S, Pondaven S, Zahrani MA, Lescanne E. Conservative management of acute mastoiditis in children. Arch Otolaryngol Head Neck Surg. 2011;137(4):346–50.

22. Groth A, Enoksson F, Stalfors J, Stenfeldt K, Hultcrantz M, Hermansson A. Recurrent acute mastoiditis—a retrospective national study in Sweden. Acta Otolaryngol. 2012;132(12):1275–81.

23. Ellefsen B, Bonding P. Facial palsy in acute otitis media. Clin Otolaryngol Allied Sci. 1996;21(5):393–5.

24. Royer M, Stott C, Rivas MP. Facial paralysis in otitis media. Literature review. Rev Otorrinolaringol Cir Cabeza Cuello. 2007;67:255–63.

25. Kitsko DJ, Dohar JE. Inner ear and facial nerve complications of acute otitis media, including vertigo. Curr Allergy Asthma Rep. 2007;7(6):444–50.

26. House JW, Brackmann DE. Facial nerve grading system. Otolaryngol Head Neck Surg. 1985 Apr;93(2):146–7.

27. Elliott CA, Zalzal GH, Gottlieb WR. Acute otitis media and facial paralysis in children. Ann Otol Rhinol Laryngol. 1996;105(1):58–62.

28. Kvestad E, Kvaerner KJ, Mair IW. Otologic facial palsy: etiology, onset, and symptom duration. Ann Otol Rhinol Laryngol. 2002;111:598–602.

29. Kamitsuka M, Feldman K, Richardson M. Facial paralysis associated with otitis media. Pediatr Infect Dis. 1985;4(6):682–4.

30. Hof E. Facial palsy of infectious origin in children. In: Fisch U, editor. Facial nerve surgery. Birmingham: Aesculapius; 1977. p. 414–418.

31. Takahashi H, Nakamura H, Yui M, Mori H. Analysis of fifty cases of facial palsy due to otitis media. Arch Otorhinolaryngol. 1985;241(2):163–8.

32. Ikeda M, Nakazato H, Onoda K, Hirai R, Kida A. Facial nerve paralysis caused by middle ear cholesteatoma and effects of surgical intervention. Acta Otolaryngol. 2006;126(1):95–100.

33. Harker LA, Pignatari SS. Facial nerve paralysis secondary to chronic otitis media without cholesteatoma. Am J Otol. 1992;13(4):372–4.

34. Altuntas A, Unal A, Aslan A, Ozcan M, Kurkcuoglu S, Nalca Y. Facial nerve paralysis in chronic suppurative otitis media: Ankara Numune Hospital experience. Auris Nasus Larynx. 1998;25(2):169–72.

35. Goldstein NA, Casselbrant ML, Bluestone CD, Kurs-Lasky M. Intratemporal complications of acute otitis media in infants and children. Otolaryngol Head Neck Surg. 1998;119(5):444–54.

36. Price T, Fayad G. Abducens nerve palsy as the sole presenting symptom of petrous apicitis. J Laryngol Otol. 2002;116(9):726–9.

37. Guedes V, et al. Gradenigo's syndrome: a case-report. Arch Argent Pediatr. 2010;108(3):e74–5.

38. Motamed M, Kalan A. Gradenigo's syndrome. Postgrad Med J. 2000;76(899):559–60.

39. Minotti AM, Kountakis SE. Management of abducens palsy in patients with petrositis. Ann Otol Rhinol Laryngol. 1999;108(9):897–902.

40. Kangsanarak J, Fooanant S, Ruckphaopunt K, Navacharoen N, Teotrakul S. Extracranial and intracranial complications of suppurative otitis media. Report of 102 cases. J Laryngol Otol. 1993;107(11):999–1004.

41. Wanna GB, Dharamsi LM, Moss JR, Bennett ML, Thompson RC, Haynes DS. Contemporary management of intracranial complications of otitis media. Otol Neurotol. 2010;31(1):111–7.

42. Migirov L, Duvdevani S, Kronenberg J. Otogenic intracranial complications: a review of 28 cases. Acta Otolaryngol. 2005;125(8):819–22.

43. Penido Nde O, Borin A, Iha LC, Suguri VM, Onishi E, Fukuda Y, Cruz OL. Intracranial complications of otitis media: 15 years of experience in 33 patients. Otolaryngol Head Neck Surg. 2005;132(1):37–42.

44. Isaacson B, Mirabal C, Kutz JW Jr, Lee KH, Roland PS. Pediatric otogenic intracranial abscesses. Otolaryngol Head Neck Surg. 2010;142(3):434–7.

45. Hafidh MA, Keogh I, Walsh RM, Walsh M, Rawluk D. Otogenic intracranial complications. a 7-year retrospective review. Am J Otolaryngol. 2006;27(6):390–5.

46. Maroldi R, Farina D, Palvarini L, Marconi A, Gadola E, Menni K, Battaglia G. Computed tomography and magnetic resonance imaging of pathologic conditions of the middle ear. Eur J Radiol. 2001;40(2):78–93.

47. Vazquez E, Castellote A, Piqueras J, Mauleon S, Creixell S, Pumarola F, et al. Imaging of complications of acute mastoiditis in children. Radiographics. 2003;23(2):359–72.

48. Slovik Y, Kraus M, Leiberman A, Kaplan DM. Role of surgery in the management of otogenic meningitis. J Laryngol Otol. 2007;121(9):897–901.

49. Wu JF, Jin Z, Yang JM, Liu YH, Duan ML. Extracranial and intracranial complications of otitis media: 22-year clinical experience and analysis. Acta Otolaryngol. 2012;132(3):261–5.

50. Dubey SP, Larawin V, Molumi CP. Intracranial spread of chronic middle ear suppuration. Am J Otolaryngol. 2010;31(2):73–7.

51. Singh B, Maharaj TJ. Radical mastoidectomy: its place in otitic intracranial complications. J Laryngol Otol. 1993;107(12):1113–8.

52. Syal R, Singh H, Duggal KK. Otogenic brain abscess: management by otologist. J Laryngol Otol. 2006;120(10):837–41. Epub 2006 Jul 6.

53. Morwani KP, Jayashankar N. Single stage, transmastoid approach for otogenic intracranial abscess. J Laryngol Otol. 2009;123(11):1216–20.

54. Au JK, Adam SI, Michaelides EM. Contemporary management of pediatric lateral sinus thrombosis: a twenty year review. Am J Otolaryngol. 2013;34(2):145–50.

55. Tov EE, Leiberman A, Shelef I, Kaplan DM. Conservative nonsurgical treatment of a child with otogenic lateral sinus thrombosis. Am J Otolaryngol. 2008;29(2):138–41. doi:10.1016/j.amjoto.2007.04.004.

56. Leibovitz E. Complicated otitis media and its implications. Vaccine. 2008;23(26 Suppl 7):G16–9.

57. Halgrimson WR, Chan KH, Abzug MJ, Perkins JN, Carosone-Link P, Simões EA. Incidence of acute mastoiditis in Colorado children in the pneumococcal conjugate vaccine era. Pediatr Infect Dis J. 2014;33(5):453–7.

58. Choi SS, Lander L. Pediatric acute mastoiditis in the post-pneumococcal conjugate vaccine era. Laryngoscope. 2011;121(5):1072–80.

59. Navazo-Eguía AI, Conejo-Moreno D, De-La-Mata-Franco G, Clemente-García A. Acute mastoiditis in the pneumococcal vaccine era. Acta Otorrinolaringol Esp. 2011;62(1):45–50.

60. Ongkasuwan J, Valdez TA, Hulten KG, Mason EO Jr, Kaplan SL. Pneumococcal mastoiditis in children and the emergence of multidrug-resistant serotype 19A isolates. Pediatrics. 2008;122(1):34–9.

Management of Otitis Media in Children Receiving Cochlear Implants

Jonathan Cavanagh and Audie Woolley

Prevalence of Meningitis and Association with Otitis Media

Interest in meningitis and its association with co-chlear implantation peaked in 2002 when it was noticed that there was a sudden increase in cases and number of fatalities in cochlear implant (CI) patients in North America and Europe. There are many known risk factors for meningitis in hearing-impaired children, but the spike in number of cases in 2002 seemed to be related to the use of a two-part electrode by one of the main CI companies. Among patients with the combination electrode and positioner CI, the incidence of meningitis was 450 cases per 100,000. This rate is much inflated from the general population incidence of meningitis of 0.5–5.0 cases per 100,000 [1].

The combination electrode and positioner CI was taken off the market by the manufacturer, but it was discovered that there were other unreported cases of meningitis with all of the most common implant manufacturers. After omitting meningitis cases associated with implants with a positioner, the incidence of meningitis was still much higher than compared to the general population, with an incidence rate of 11–14 cases per 100,000 [2].

There are a number of reasons why CI patients are at an increased risk of developing meningitis, an increase which is elevated during the first 2 months after implantation. It has been postulated that bacteria causing meningitis in CI patients enter through the middle and inner ear [3]. From these locations hematogenous dissemination and a process of osteothrombophlebitis represent possible routes of infection spread from the middle ear to intra- or extracranial locations. Postulated pathways include the oval or round window, development of dehiscence of the floor of the hypotympanum, or from previous ear surgery [4]. There are also factors independent of cochlear implantation which may place children with hearing loss at increased risk of bacterial meningitis [5]. Inner ear malformations are more common in children with hearing loss, which also increases their risk of developing bacterial meningitis [6–9]. In a case-control study, the combination of radiographic evidence of an inner ear malformation and a cerebrospinal fluid (CSF) leak was associated with an increased risk of all subtypes of meningitis, and the presence of a CSF leak alone was associated with an increased risk of perioperative meningitis [3]. Preimplant meningitis has been identified as a risk factor for postimplant meningitis [10]. In a study in Denmark, it was found that in young children with hearing loss (10.4 % of the cohort had CIs), the rate of meningitis was 43 cases per 100,000 person-years [11].

J. Cavanagh (✉)
Department of Surgery, Janeway Children's Hospital,
300 Prince Philip Drive St John's, Newfoundland,
Canada
e-mail: jpcnfld@gmail.com

A. Woolley
Department of Otolaryngology and Pediatrics, The
Children's Hospital of Alabama, Birmingham, AL, USA
e-mail: Audie.Woolley@childrensal.org

© Springer International Publishing Switzerland 2015
D. Preciado (ed.), *Otitis Media: State of the art concepts and treatment*, DOI 10.1007/978-3-319-17888-2_14

The study determined that children with hearing loss were found to have a three- to fivefold increased risk for developing meningitis. Another important factor in the increased risk of developing meningitis in CI patients is the trend toward earlier placement of implants, due to improved development of speech and language with earlier implantation [12–14]. Widespread screening of newborn hearing identifies children for implantation at a time when their risk of developing meningitis is the highest [15]. In Rubin and Papsin's paper [16] on prevention and treatment of acute otitis media (AOM) and meningitis in CI patients the authors advocate that all implant candidates be immunized with age-appropriate doses of pneumococcal conjugate, Haemophilus influenza type b conjugate vaccines, and appropriate annual immunization against influenza. Also, as a preventative measure against meningitis, children at the age of two should have a single dose of the 23-valent pneumococcal polysaccharide vaccine (Table 14.1) [17].

Aggressiveness of Otitis Media Diagnosis and Treatment

The usual age of cochlear implantation in children corresponds to the peak age for the development of AOM [1, 2]. Teele et al. [18] reported that by 1 year of age, 62 % of the children had one or more episodes of AOM, and 17 % had three or more episodes of AOM. By 3 years of age, 83 % had one or more episodes of AOM, and 46 % had three or more episodes of AOM. This can be explained by the anatomy and physiology of the Eustachian tube of a young child and the surrounding lymphoepithelial ring that can prevent adequate drainage of the middle ear in childhood [18]. Of concern is the belief that children with CIs may be more susceptible to the complications of otitis media (OM) due to the surgical violation of the cochlea, the presence of a foreign body in the inner ear, and the potential for spread from a purulent middle ear through the cochleostomy to the CSF via the inner ear.

In a retrospective review of 234 patients who underwent cochlear implantation, it was found that children with a preimplantation history of AOM had a higher risk of postimplantation AOM than healthy children with CIs [19]; but this risk

Table 14.1 Recommended pneumococcal vaccination schedule for persons with CIs [34]

Age at first PCV7 dose (months)[a]	PCV7 primary series	PCV7 additional dose	PPV23 dose
2–6	3 doses, 2 months apart[b]	1 dose at 12–15 months of age[e]	Indicated at 24 months of age[f]
7–11	2 doses, 2 months apart[b]	1 dose at 12–15 months of age[e]	Indicated at 24 months of age[f]
12–23	2 doses, 2 months apart[c]	Not indicated	Indicated at 24 months of age[f]
24–59	2 doses, 2 month apart[c]	Not indicated	Indicated[f]
≥60	Not indicated[d]	Not indicated[d]	Indicated

PCV7 7-valent pneumococcal conjugate vaccine, *PPV23* 23-valent pneumococcal polysaccharide vaccine
[a] A schedule with a reduced number of total PCV7 doses is indicated if children start late or are incompletely vaccinated. Children with a lapse in vaccination should be vaccinated according to the catch-up schedule [32]
[b] For children vaccinated at age <1 year, the minimum interval between doses is 4 weeks
[c] Minimum interval between doses is 8 weeks
[d] PCV7 is not recommended for children aged ≥5 years
[e] The additional dose should be administered 8 weeks after the primary series has been completed
[f] Children aged <5 years should complete the PCV7 series first; 23-valent PPV23 should be administered to children 24 months of age 8 weeks after the last dose of PCV7 [33]

does seem to decrease after cochlear implantation [19, 20, 21]. More than half of the children who suffered from AOM after cochlear implantation had no history of AOM prior to implantation [19].

There is debate as to how aggressive the treatment of AOM should be in CI patients. Four retrospective studies [19, 22–24] of AOM in children with implants have been conducted. In three studies, the treatment of the AOM was found to be satisfactory when using standard treatments of systemic antimicrobial therapy with initial empiric treatment with an oral antimicrobial agent (e.g., amoxicillin at a dose of 80–90 mg/kg per day). In contrast, the fourth study [24] revealed that patients with implants were more likely to require intravenous antimicrobial therapy and a myringotomy. Of the 11 episodes of AOM reported in this fourth study, 7 patients underwent surgical treatment for mastoiditis. No child in any of the four series was reported to have developed bacterial meningitis. The immediate postoperative period appears to be a sensitive time for the potential development of meningitis. For this reason, AOM in the immediate postoperative period demands aggressive treatment. Rubin and Papsin [16] recommend that AOM diagnosed during the first 2 months after implantation be initially treated with parenteral antibiotics (e.g., ceftriaxone or cefotaxime).

Watchful waiting is inappropriate for CI patients as the presence of such a large foreign body, with the increased risk of meningitis even without a prior history of AOM, makes the prompt use of antibiotics mandatory [25]. There are certain circumstances in which a CI patient would be at higher risk for developing meningitis. Those risk factors include: (1) The CI has a space/positioner (Advanced Bionics model AB-5100H or AB-5100H-11); (2) the episode occurs within the first 2 months of implantation; (3) the patient has a known inner malformation or CSF/middle ear fistula; (4) the patient appears severely ill with evidence of mastoiditis or inner ear infection [16]. In such circumstances, a middle ear aspirate should be sought immediately for culture and sensitivity to antibiotics. Based on clinical judgment and culture results, the physician can decide on the mode of antibiotic treatment

(oral vs. intravenous), which antibiotics to use, and whether or not to hospitalize the patient [26]. Implant patients with a middle ear effusion or an AOM along with suspected meningitis should have both CSF and a middle ear aspirate sent for culture and sensitivity. If presenting in the first 2 months after implantation, antimicrobials should include coverage against gram-negative bacilli (e.g., meropenum) plus vancomycin [16].

Role of Tympanostomy Tubes

Traditionally it was thought that disruption of the tympanic membrane with a foreign body in the middle ear could pose a potential risk for dangerous seeding of the CI. This theory likely arises from stapedectomy surgery where, like cochlear implantation, the inner ear is opened, and it is felt ideal to perform such surgery in a "sterile" middle ear with an intact tympanic membrane. However, children frequently arrive for their initial CI assessment with myringotomy tubes (MTs) in place. The MTs may have been placed for a middle ear effusion to ensure an adequate hearing aid trial, or they may have been placed for recurrent OM [27].

In a survey of CI surgeons [28], 56% of respondents stated that they would proceed with cochlear implantation with MTs in place if the ears were clean and dry. The majority of the remaining respondents stated that they would remove the tube and wait for the tympanic membrane perforation to heal. However, as Kennedy and Shelton noted in their study [28], this choice of action may be fraught with difficulty—the tympanic membrane may fail to heal spontaneously, or fluid or infection may return behind the tympanic membrane. Such situations would undoubtedly cause anxiety, frustration, and delay for the patient and caregivers. Also, early implantation is vital to take advantage of the plasticity of hearing development in young children, and unnecessary delay should be avoided [29].

The American Academy of Pediatrics approved the judicious use of MTs in CI candidates. A policy statement was issued [16] on the management of OM in CI patients which states that surgeons should manage OM with MT placement either before or at the time of cochlear implantation to prevent further OM episodes.

In the event that a child with a CI develops OM while an MT is in place, a sample culture can be taken, and the patient should be started on systemic and topical antibiotics as well as local otorrhea care [26].

For those patients who develop recurrent bouts of AOM with a CI in place, it has been argued that the indications for MTs and their management in the CI recipients should be the same as those in the patients without a CI. MTs should be placed in any CI patient having recurrent bouts of AOM. There does not appear to be an issue having a CI and MTs in place if warranted [27].

Implant with Middle Ear Effusions

The question as to whether MTs should be placed in CI patients with a persistent middle ear effusion post implantation remains unanswered as there is limited research in this area.

In the study completed by Yin [30], a review of 186 children with CIs had discovered four cases of persistent middle ear effusions occurring after implantation. The effusions cleared in two patients after 2 weeks of intravenous antibiotics. The other two children who presented with unilateral, repeated OM with effusion despite intravenous antibiotic treatment were treated with MTs. The authors advocated against an observation period without antibiotic treatment for these patients. They suggested aggressive treatment of the middle ear for children with CIs to prevent the development of a retraction pocket, adhesion of tympanic membrane, and cholesteatoma formation [30]. It is our policy in dealing with chronic middle ear effusions in preoperative candidates for a CI to go ahead by placing an MT in those children and proceeding with the CI while the MT is in place. If an effusion is noted at the time of CI surgery, cochlear implantation is carried out and an MT is placed at the same time. If a child has a persistent middle ear effusion of longer than 6 weeks after cochlear implantation,

then an MT is placed. If an AOM is noted at the time of CI surgery, the surgery is delayed until resolution of the infection.

Future Research

As of 2010, approximately 219,000 patients worldwide have received implants, and with changing indications to allow more patients to benefit from cochlear implantation, it is increasingly likely that a primary care physician will have a patient in their practice with an implant [31]. It is therefore imperative that otolaryngologists as well as primary care providers be familiar with the treatment of AOM in CI patients. Patients as well should be educated regarding the signs and symptoms of infections including AOM, mastoiditis, meningitis, and the need for appropriate vaccinations preoperatively. Early treatment can prevent implant malfunction and more serious complications of these infections.

References

1. Biernath KR, Reefhuis J, Whitney CG, et al. Bacterial meningitis among children with cochlear implants beyond 24 months after implantation. Pediatrics. 2006;117(2):284–9.
2. Cohen NL. Does meningitis after cochlear implantation remain a concern in 2011? Otol Neurotol. 2012;33(1):93–5.
3. Reefhuis J, Honein MA, Whitney CG, et al. Risk of bacterial meningitis in children with cochlear implants. N Engl J Med. 2003;349:435–45.
4. Neely JG. Complications of temporal bone infection. In: Cummings CW, Fredrickson JM, Harker LA, Krause CJ, Schuller DE, editors. Otolaryngology-head and neck surgery, vol. 4, second ed. St. Louis: Mosby-Year Book, Inc.; 1993. p 2840–5.
5. Arnold W, Bredberg G, Gstöttner W, et al. Meningitis following cochlear implantation: pathomechanisms, clinical symptoms, conservative and surgical treatments. ORL J Otorhinolaryngol Relat Spec. 2002;64(6):382–9.
6. Herther C, Schindler RA. Mondini's dysplasia with recurrent meningitis. Laryngoscope. 1985;95:655–8.
7. Hayashi N, Kino M, Nobori U, et al. Recurrent bacterial meningitis: secondary to malformation of the inner ear. Clin Pediatr (Phila). 1989;28:139–41.
8. Phelps PD, King A, Michaels L. Cochlear dysplasia and meningitis. Am J Otol 1994;15: 551–7.

9. Valmari P, Palva A. Recurrent meningitis due to pneumococci and non-typable *Haemophilus influenzae* in a child with a *Mondini malformation*. Infection. 1986;14:36–7.

10. FDA. FDA Public Health Web Notification: cochlear implant recipients may be at greater risk for meningitis. July 24, 2002; updated August 15, 2002, and October 17m 2002. www.fda.gov/cdrh/safety/cochlear.html. Accessed 17 Oct 2002.

11. Parner ET, Reefhuis J, Schendel D, Thomsen JL, Ovesen T, Thorsen P. Hearing loss diagnosis followed by meningitis in Danish children, 1995–2004. Otolaryngol Head Neck Surg. 2007;136(3):428–33.

12. Hammes DM, Novak MA, Rotz LA, Willis M, Edmondson DM, Thomas JF. Early identification and cochlear implantation: critical factors for spoken language development. Ann Otol Rhinol Laryngol Suppl. 2002;189:74–8.

13. Govaerts PJ, De Beukelaer C, Daemers K, et al. Outcome of cochlear implantation at different ages from 0 to 6 years. Otol Neurotol. 2002;23:885–90.

14. Sharma A, Dorman And MF, Spahr AJ. A sensitive period for the development of the central auditory system in children with cochlear implants: implications for age of implantation. Ear Hear. 2002;23:532–9.

15. Schuchat A, Robinson K, Wenger JD, et al. Bacterial meningitis in the United States in 1995. N Engl J Med. 1997;337:970–6.

16. Rubin LG, Papsin B. Cochlear implants in children: surgical site infections and prevention and treatment of acute otitis media and meningitis. Committee on Infectious Diseases and Section on Otolaryngology-Head and Neck Surgery. Pediatrics. 2010;126(2):381–91.

17. Centers for Disease Control and Prevention (CDC). Pneumococcal vaccination for cochlear implant recipients. MMWR. 2002;51:931.

18. Teele DW, Klein JO, Rosner B. Epidemiology of otitis media during the first seven years of life in children in great Boston: a prospective, cohort study. J Infect Dis. 1989;160:83–94.

19. Migirov L, Yakirevitch A, Henkin Y, Kaplan-Neeman R, Kronenberg J. Acute otitis media and mastoiditis following cochlear implantation. Int J Pediatr Otorhinolaryngol. 2006;70(5):899–903.

20. Luntz M, Teszler CB, Shpak T, et al. Cochlear implantation in healthy and otitis-prone children; a prospective study. Laryngoscope. 2001;111:1614–18.

21. Luntz M, Hodges AV, Balkany T, et al. Otitis media in children with cochlear implants. Laryngoscope. 1996;106:1403–1405.

22. House WF, Berliner KI, Eisenberg LS. Experiences with the cochlear implant in preschool children. Ann Otol Rhinol Laryngol. 1983;92(6 pt 1):587–92.

23. House WF, Luxford WM, Courtney B. Otitis media in children following the cochlear implant. Ear Hear. 1985;6(3 suppl):24S–6S.

24. Kempf HG, Stöver T, Lenarz T. Mastoiditis and acute otitis media in children with cochlear implants: recommendations for medical management. Ann Otol Rhinol Laryngol Suppl. 2000;185:25–7.

25. American Academy of Pediatrics. Subcommittee on management of acute otitis media. Diagnosis and management of acute otitis media. Pediatrics. 2004;113(5):1451–65.

26. Luntz M, Teszler CB, Shpak T. Cochlear implantation in children with otitis media: second stage of a long-term prospective study. Int J Pediatr Otorhinolaryngol. 2004;68(3):273–80.

27. Barañano CF, Sweitzer RS, Mahalak ML, Alexander NS, Woolley AL. The management of myringotomy tubes in pediatric cochlear implant recipients. Arch Otolaryngol Head Neck Surg. 2010;136(6):557–60.

28. Kennedy RJ, Shelton C. Ventilation tubes and cochlear implants what do we do? Otol Neurotol. 2005;26(3):438–41.

29. Cheng AK, Grant GD, Niparko JK. Meta-analysis of pediatric cochlear implant literature. Ann Otol Rhinol Laryngol. 1999;177:124–8.

30. Lin YS. Management of otitis media-related diseases in children with a cochlear implant. Acta Otolaryngol. 2009;129(3):254–60.

31. National Institute on Deafness and Other Communication Disorders, National Institutes of Health. Cochlear implants. www.nidcd.nih.gov/health/hearing/coch.asp. Accessed Aug 2014.

32. Centers for Disease Control and Prevention (CDC). Pneumococcal conjugate vaccine shortage resolved. MMWR. 2003;52:446–7.

33. Centers for Disease Control and Prevention (CDC). Preventing pneumococcal disease among infants and young children: recommendations of the Advisory Committee on Immunization Practices (ACIP). MMWR Recomm Rep. 2000;49(RR-9):1–38.

34. Centers for Disease Control and Prevention, Advisory Committee on Immunization Practices. Pneumococcal vaccination for cochlear implant candidates and recipients: updated recommendations of the Advisory Committee on Infectious Practices. MMWR Morb Mortal Wkly Rep. 2003;52(31):739–740.

Index

© Springer International Publishing Switzerland 2015
D. Preciado (ed.), *Otitis Media: State of the art concepts and treatment,* DOI 10.1007/978-3-319-17888-2

Printed by Printforce, the Netherlands